Wanderson Pereira
Mário Roberto Hatayde

Experimental Cupric Poisoning in Sheep

Wanderson Pereira
Mário Roberto Hatayde

Experimental Cupric Poisoning in Sheep

Clinical and Laboratory Aspects

ScienciaScripts

Imprint
Any brand names and product names mentioned in this book are subject to trademark, brand or patent protection and are trademarks or registered trademarks of their respective holders. The use of brand names, product names, common names, trade names, product descriptions etc. even without a particular marking in this work is in no way to be construed to mean that such names may be regarded as unrestricted in respect of trademark and brand protection legislation and could thus be used by anyone.

Cover image: www.ingimage.com

This book is a translation from the original published under ISBN 978-613-9-63074-5.

Publisher:
Sciencia Scripts
is a trademark of
Dodo Books Indian Ocean Ltd. and OmniScriptum S.R.L publishing group

120 High Road, East Finchley, London, N2 9ED, United Kingdom
Str. Armeneasca 28/1, office 1, Chisinau MD-2012, Republic of Moldova, Europe
Printed at: see last page
ISBN: 978-620-7-76606-2

SUMMARY

DEDICATORY 3

EXPERIMENTAL CRYPTIC INTOXICATION IN SHEEP: CLINICAL AND LABORATORY ASPECTS. 4

1. INTRODUCTION AND LITERATURE REVIEW 5

2. BACKGROUND 9

3. OBJECTIVES 10

4. MATERIAL AND METHODS 11

5. RESULTS 15

6. Discussion 46

7. CONCLUSION 51

8. BIBLIOGRAPHICAL REFERENCES 52

APPENDIX 1 56

"There are men who fight one day and are good.

There are others who fight for a year and are better.

There are those who fight for many years and are very good.

But there are those who fight all their lives.

Those are the essentials. "

Bertolt Brecht

DEDICATORY

To my grandparents,

Jûlio José Biscola and Jûlia Vieira Biscola

Examples of strength and faith to follow!

To my parents,

Wanderley Aparecido Pereira and Maria Sônia Biscola Pereira

The basis of my achievements!

My beloved wife,

Joice Lara Maia Faria

My reason for living!

To my children, Jûlia and Bruno

The future of my existence!

For their affection, love, example, encouragement and understanding....

If today I have reached another milestone, it is because you believed in my success and walked by my side.

THANK YOU VERY MUCH!!!

EXPERIMENTAL CRYPTIC INTOXICATION IN SHEEP: CLINICAL AND LABORATORY ASPECTS.

SUMMARY - Sheep have a tendency to accumulate copper in the body. When the liver's storage capacity is exhausted, copper is released into the blood causing clinical signs of intoxication. In order to verify the changes in serum biochemistry, blood count, erythrocyte morphology, serum protein profile and serum copper concentration during the pre-hemolytic and hemolytic phases of chronic copper intoxication, six sheep were randomly divided into two groups: G-1 (control) and G-2 (experimentally intoxicated). In addition to the daily diet, the three sheep in G-2 received 3mg of $CuSO_4$. $5H_2O$/Kg BW, followed by weekly increases of 3mg of $CuSO_4$. $5H_2O$/ Kg BW in the daily dose. The sheep in both groups were examined daily. To obtain the blood count and biochemical blood components, samples were taken before (M0 - M3), during (M4) and after (M5 and M6) the hemolytic crisis. Necropsies were carried out on the G-2 sheep that died and the G-1 sheep that were euthanized at the end of the experiment and fragments of their liver were taken for histopathological evaluation. During the pre-hemolytic phase, there were few alterations, but during the hemolytic crisis, the G-2 sheep showed normochromic macrocytic anemia, a predominance of red blood cells with acanthocyte morphology, leukocytosis with neutrophilia, elevated serum AST, GGT and CK levels and hypercupremia; serum ceruloplasmin levels were reduced and the levels of transferrin, protein of 35.The intoxicated animals had anorexia, icteric mucous membranes, soft, dark green feces and hemoglobinuria. Necropsy revealed yellowish mucous membranes, liver and other tissues, blackened kidneys and brownish urine. Liver histopathology showed hepatocyte megalocytosis, disorganization of hepatocyte cords, cholestasis and peri-portal lymphocytic inflammatory infiltrate.

Keywords: copper, sheep, intoxication, red blood cells, scanning electron microscopy, ceruloplasmin.

1. INTRODUCTION AND LITERATURE REVIEW

In addition to organic molecules, animal tissues also contain inorganic molecules which account for around 2 to 5% of the animal's total weight. Among these elements, minerals have essential functions both in the structure of tissues and biomolecules, and in metabolism itself, participating as enzyme co-factors, hormone activators, and as responsible for osmotic pressure and acid-base balance (GONZALEZ et al., 2000).

Among the minerals, copper (Cu) is an essential element for animal survival as it acts as a component of many metalloproteins such as ceruloplasmin, superoxide dismutase (CuZnSOD) and cytochrome oxidase (McDOWELL, 1992; UNDERWOOD & SUTTLE, 2001; BRADBERRY, 2007; ZHANG, et. al., 2008).

After ingestion, copper is absorbed mainly in the small intestine and its transport through the intestinal mucosa is controlled by a metalloprotein called metallothionein. The higher its concentration, the lower the absorption of copper (ORTOLANI, 2002). After passing through the intestinal mucosa, copper binds to albumin and is transported via the hepatic portal circulation to the liver to be incorporated into ceruloplasmin and then reach the systemic circulation and distributed throughout the body (BRADBERRY, 2007).

Copper deficiency and toxicity in ruminants occur frequently in many parts of the world (MILTIMORE & MASON, 1971). The development of copper deficiency or excess depends on both the concentration of this element in the diet and the concentrations of antagonists that interfere with absorption and subsequent utilization for metabolic processes (GOONERATNE et al., 1989).

Among animal species, sheep are the most prone to both copper deficiency and copper poisoning (ORTOLANI, 1996; GOONERATNE et al., 1989). Deficiency is linked to the lower capacity of some sheep breeds to absorb copper, while copper poisoning is due to a lower capacity for conjugation between copper and metallothionein, reducing the excretion of this element from the body via the bile duct and allowing it to accumulate in the liver (SOARES, 2004).

Concentrations of 20 to 110 mg of Cu/kg of dry matter (DM) in sheep are sufficient to cause acute poisoning, while ingestion of 3.5 mg of Cu/kg of body weight (BW), with levels in the diet ranging from 20 to 25 ppm, is responsible for causing chronic poisoning (RADOSTITS et al., 2002; SMITH, 2006). HUMANN-ZIEHANK & BICKHARDT (2001), using a concentration of 3.7 mg of Cu/kg of body weight for 84 days, found no clinical signs of intoxication. SANSINANEA et al. (1996) induced cupric intoxication in sheep using

10ml/kg of body weight of a 2% solution of copper sulphate pentahydrate ($CuSO_4. 5 H_2O$) for five days a week and found signs of intoxication from the 12th week onwards, with hemolysis during the 15th week. SOARES (2004), obtained symptoms of chronic intoxication between 30 and 96 days with a dose of 3 mg/Kg B.C./day, adding 3mg/Kg B.C. to the daily dose every week.

Copper accumulation can occur in three circumstances: primary intoxication caused by ingesting excessive amounts of Cu; secondary phytogenic intoxication, in which, despite Cu being ingested in normal quantities, the microelement accumulates as a result of low molybdenum levels; secondary hepatogenic poisoning, in which Cu, ingested at normal levels, accumulates in the liver as a result of liver damage caused by plants containing pyrrolizidine alkaloids (RIET-CORREA et al., 1989).

Copper intoxication can be divided into two forms: acute intoxication, resulting from the abrupt ingestion of large amounts of copper in a short space of time; and accumulative copper intoxication, where the accumulation of hepatic copper is progressive and can last from months to years, until the onset of the hemolytic phase (ORTOLANI et al., 2003).

Chronic copper poisoning can be divided into three distinct phases: pre-hemolytic, hemolytic and post-hemolytic. During the pre-hemolytic phase, copper accumulates in the liver without any clinical signs appearing. Copper accumulates initially in the perivenous hepatocytes and later in other areas of the liver.

During accumulation, hepatocytes considerably increase their number of isosomes, an organelle in which copper also accumulates. Once the maximum accumulation threshold is reached, diffuse cell death occurs, promoting the significant release of copper and lysozymes. The free copper moves into the bloodstream, where after entering the red blood cells it oxidizes glutathione, the substance responsible for the integrity of these cells, culminating in hemolysis around 24 hours later (ORTOLANI, 1996).

During the hemolytic crisis, neutrophilia and anemia are observed. Há increased blood levels of copper and serum levels of sorbitol dehydrogenase (SDH), arginase, aspartate amino transferase (AST), glutamate dehydrogenase (GD), ceruloplasmin, urea and bilirubin (MÉNDEZ, 2001). An acute hemolytic crisis with hemoglobinemia and hemoglobinuria are important findings. Heinz corpuscles can be found in stained red blood cells in blood smears (INABA, 2000).

Death can result from severe liver and kidney damage and the degree of anemia. Animals rarely survive the clinical picture characteristic of a hemolytic crisis (KOWALCZYK et al.

1964; MÉNDEZ, 2001). Those that do survive recover slowly over the course of two to three weeks during the post-hemolytic phase (ORTOLANI, 1996).

The mechanism of hemolysis caused by copper intoxication is not well understood. According to JAIN (1993) and INABA (2000), the cytotoxic effects occur due to the interaction of copper with a series of compounds present in the erythrocyte membranes, generating the formation of oxidizing agents in this process, as well as the inhibition of important enzymes for red blood cells such as glutathione reductase and pyruvate kinase, leading to an increase in the formation of methemoglobin. The direct action of superoxide anions and hydrogen peroxide inside erythrocytes culminates in the formation of Heinz bodies.

The clinical picture varies. In the acute form, abdominal pain, intense thirst, diarrhea and the presence of hypercolic stools stand out. In the accumulative form, hemoglobinuria, jaundice, tachypnea and the presence of chocolate-colored episcleral vessels are noteworthy. In both clinical forms, death can occur in around 30 to 40 hours (ORTOLANI, 1996; MÉNDEZ, 2001).

The diagnosis can be made using the history, clinical signs, laboratory tests and necropsy findings. Values higher than 800 ppm Cu/Kg DM in the liver and 100 ppm Cu/Kg DM in the kidney are considered conclusive (RIET- CORREA et al., 1989; ORTOLANI, 1996; LEMOS et al., 1997; MÉNDEZ, 2001). Analysis of copper in the diet is also recommended. The dosage of AST and GGT, together with the serum copper concentration are the main biochemical tests for the diagnosis and monitoring of copper poisoning (AUZA, et al., 1999), as well as the dosage of alkaline phosphatase (ALP) (TURK & CASTEEL, 1997), since the enzymes that indicate liver damage can be elevated 4 to 6 weeks before the hemolytic crisis (MÉNDEZ, 2001). AST is the first enzyme proposed to identify chronic copper poisoning. An increase in GGT levels indicates very old damage to the bile ducts (UNDERWOOD & SUTTLE, 2001). According to TENNANT (1997), liver function should be determined by measuring the enzymes AST, GGT and ALP, which indicate the presence of acute or chronic liver damage.

Necropsy of the animals revealed macroscopic lesions characterized by generalized jaundice, serous fluid in the peritoneal, thoracic and pericardial cavities, a friable yellow or orange liver, dark brown, swollen kidneys and dark red urine. In the liver, hepatocytes are enlarged, pleomorphic and have vacuoles of various sizes in their cytoplasm. Some nuclei are on the periphery of the hepatocytes, in others the chromatin is marginalized and intranuclear vacuoles can be seen. Bile can be seen in the bile ducts. In the portal space there is proliferation of bile duct cells, proliferation of fibrous tissue and infiltration of inflammatory cells. The Kupffer cells have a yellowish brown pigment. In the kidney, the tubules show reddish hyaline or granular cylinders. Interstitial fibroplasia can be seen. The kidney lesions are caused by the accumulation of copper in the epithelial cells, associated with the hypercupremia and hemoglobinuria that occur during the hemolytic crisis (BOSTWICK, 1982; RIET-CORREA et al., 1989; LEMOS, et al., 1997; MÉNDEZ, 2001).

Therapy consists of the immediate removal of the copper-rich diet. It is recommended to administer 3.4 mg of ammonium tetrathiomolybidate/kg body weight. Treated animals show rapid clinical improvement, significantly reducing serum copper levels and the activity of enzymes that indicate liver function, as well as stopping hemolysis (HUMPHRIES et al., 1988; ORTOLANI, 1996; AUZA et al., 1999; SOARES, 2004).

This intoxication must be controlled, especially when using sheep of more susceptible breeds, such as Sulffolk and Texel, and in stabled animals that receive concentrates for long periods. In these cases, it is recommended that dietary copper levels do not exceed 10 ppm, the forage/concentrate ratio does not decrease from 60:40 and mineral supplements do not contain more than 800 ppm of copper (ORTOLANI, 1996).

2. BACKGROUND

Cupric intoxication is an important fact to consider in sheep farming, since the productive demands of genetic selection and intensive management systems have increased the risk of nutritional imbalances and metabolic diseases in the flock (GONZALEZ et al., 2000).

Sheep have a tendency to accumulate copper in the body, so the use of concentrates in their diet can lead to a serious increase in liver copper levels, so that in stressful situations, or when the liver's storage capacity is exhausted, copper is rapidly released into the blood, causing poisoning (GONZALEZ et al., 2000).

This disease is of great importance because the vast majority of animals affected are of high genetic potential and economic value, and the lethality of untreated animals is over 80% (ORTOLANI, 1996).

3. OBJECTIVES

•   To evaluate liver function by determining the serum activity of the enzymes AST, GGT and CK in the pre-hemolytic, hemolytic and post-hemolytic phases of intoxicated animals;

•   Obtain the blood count of the experimentally intoxicated animals in the intoxication phases and the control group, visualizing the erythrocyte morphology in scanning electron microscopy (SEM);

•   To detect, with the aid of optical microscopy, changes in the liver parenchyma of intoxicated sheep after the hemolytic phase of intoxication;

•   Identify the serum protein profile in polyacrylamide gel electrophoresis (SDS-PAGE) of sheep in the intoxication phases and the control group;

•   Determine the serum concentration of copper in the blood serum of the animals in the intoxication phase and in the control group.

4. MATERIAL AND METHODS

4.1. Animals and Facilities

Six adult, clean, castrated sheep of no defined breed were used, housed individually in metabolic cages equipped with plastic feeders and drinkers, located in a covered area next to the Research Support Laboratory of the Veterinary Clinic and Surgery Department of the Faculty of Agricultural and Veterinary Sciences/ UNESP/ Jaboticabal *Campus* (FCAV/ UNESP). Before the experiment began, the sheep, which were grazing *Brachiaria decumbens* grass, underwent a fifteen-day adaptation period. During this period, in addition to the diet, the animals were de-wormed with albendazole (15 mg/kg body weight).

4.2. Food and nutrition

The animals were given a daily diet consisting of 700g of dry matter of Tifton 85 hay (*Cynodon* spp), water at will and 200g of concentrate[1] . The feed was subjected to bromatological analysis before the start of the experiment, checking mainly the concentrations of copper, molybdenum and sulphur (Appendix 1).

4.3. Design and induction model for cumulative copper intoxication

The animals were randomly divided into two groups (G-1 and G-2) of three animals:

- G-1: three sheep that received only the diet mentioned in item 4.2 (control);

- G-2: three sheep that received the G-1 diet + 3mg $CuSO_4$. $5H2O^2$ / Kg BW/ day, in a 5% aqueous solution, orally, with the help of a syringe, in the first week, followed by weekly increases of 3mg $CuSO_4$. $5H2O$/ Kg BW in the daily dose, following the recommendations of Soares (2004) until the appearance of macroscopic hemoglobinuria.

Blood samples were taken at the following times to obtain the blood count and the biochemical components of the blood serum:

M0 - Baseline moment;

M1 - ± 30 days before the hemolytic crisis;

M2 - ± 15 days before the hemolytic crisis;

M3 - ± 7 days before the hemolytic crisis;

M4 - Day of the hemolytic crisis;

---

1 Nutriovinos - PURINA - Brazil.
2 Copper sulphate pentahydrate - VETEC.

M5 - 24 hours after the hemolytic crisis;

M6 - 48 hours after hemolytic crisis.

4.4. Physical examination

A physical examination of the sheep in G-1 and G-2 was carried out daily. The examination began by inspecting the animals from a distance, evaluating their behavior, attitude and posture and comparing the intoxicated animals with those in the control group. Sheep that showed some kind of alteration on inspection were subjected to a more detailed physical examination with an assessment of rectal temperature, heart rate, respiratory rate, mucous membrane color and rumen motility.

4.5. Collection of biological material

4.5.1. Blood samples

The blood samples were taken in 2 sterilized and siliconized tubes[3] , duly identified, one with a capacity of 4.5 mL, containing ethylene diamine tetraacetic acid (EDTA) as an anticoagulant and the other, without anticoagulant, with a capacity of 10 mL for obtaining whole blood and serum, respectively.

The samples containing anticoagulant were promptly refrigerated, taken to the laboratory and used for blood count, blood smear and scanning electron microscopy. The samples without anticoagulant were centrifuged for 10 minutes at 3000 rpm and the serum aliquots were placed in tubes with a capacity of 2,000 μL[4] and stored at - 20°C. They were used to carry out biochemical tests and serum copper levels.

4.5.2. Fig fragments

The liver fragments were obtained during necropsy, immediately after the death of the experimentally intoxicated animals and after the euthanasia of the animals in the control group. After collection, the liver specimens were placed in vials containing 10% neutral, phosphate-buffered formaldehyde for histopathological examinations.

4.6. Analytical methods

4.6.1.. Blood samples (serum and whole blood).

4.6.1.1.   Complete blood count

The total leukocyte and red blood cell count was carried out manually by diluting the

---

3Vacutainer®
4 Eppendorf®

samples for counting in the Neubauer chamber. For the RBC count, a 1:200 dilution was made in 0.9% NaCl solution, while the leukocyte count was made in a 1:50 dilution in RBC lysing solution.

Hemoglobin values were determined by the colorimetric method, using a set of commercial reagents[5] , which were read on the semi-automatic biochemical analyzer LABQUEST[6] at a wavelength appropriate to the parameter analyzed.

The globular volume was obtained in 75 mm capillary tubes, where the samples were centrifuged at 13,000 rpm for 5 minutes and then read on a microhematocrit chart.

The hematimetric indices, mean corpuscular volume (MCV) and mean corpuscular hemoglobin concentration (MCHC) were calculated using the equations described by JAIN (1993).

Differential leukocyte counts were obtained on blood smears, stained by Rosenfeld, under a common optical microscope (THRALL, 2007).

4.6.1.2. Scanning Electron Microscopy

To assess erythrocyte morphology, blood samples containing EDTA were prepared for SEM. For this, 100 µl of blood were placed in 1.5% glutaraldehyde in 0.1M phosphate buffer, pH 7.4. After fixation for one hour at 4°C, the cells were washed three times with phosphate buffer (0.1M and pH 7.4), dehydrated in an ascending series of acetone (25 to 100%), remaining 15 minutes in each solution and with two passes in absolute acetone. Subsequently, the cells were suspended again in 100 µl of absolute acetone; two drops of this suspension were placed on a glass coverslip and quickly dried by evaporation. The coverslips were covered with a thin layer of gold (15nm)[7] and examined using a scanning electron microscope[8] at an angle of 33 to 45 degrees negative and a voltage of 15 kV, with the best fields being photographed.

4.6.1.3. Serum biochemistry

Liver function was assessed by determining the activities of the enzymes aspartate aminotransferase - AST (UV-IFCC method), gamma glutamyl transferase - GGT (modified Szasz method) using sets of commercial LABTEST reagents with readings taken on a LABQUEST semi-automatic biochemical analyzer at wavelengths appropriate to the parameters analyzed. To determine the activity of the creatine kinase enzyme, a dry

---

5 Labtest, Belo Horizonte - MG
6 Labquest, Labtest, Belo Horizonte - MG
7 DESK-II Metallizer - DENTON VACCUM
8 JSM5410 - JEOL

biochemistry technique was used, with readings taken on a Reflotron biochemical analyzer.[9]

4.6.1.3.1 Serum proteinogram.

Total protein levels (Biuret method) were obtained using sets of commercial reagents[4] ; readings were taken on a LABQUEST5 semi-automatic biochemical analyzer at the appropriate wavelength. Protein fractionation was carried out using sodium dodecyl sulfate-acrylamide gel electrophoresis (SDS-PAGE), according to the technique described by LAEMMLI (1970). After fractionation, the gel was stained for 10 min in a solution of coomassie blue and then placed in a solution of 7% acetic acid to remove the excess dye, until the protein fractions were clear. The concentrations of these proteins were determined using a computerized densitometer[10] . As a reference, we used the marker solution[11] with molecular weights of 29,000, 45,000, 66,000, 97,400, 116,000 and 205,000 daltons (Da), as well as purified proteins[7] - albumin, IgG, haptoglobin, α_1-antitrypsin and transferrin.

4.6.1.3.2 Determination of serum copper levels

The serum copper content was determined by diluting the serum sample twenty times in 0.1N HCl (200µL of serum and 1,800µL of HCl) and reading it using atomic absorption spectrophotometry (KARGIN et al., 2004).

4.6.2. Histological examination

The liver samples collected during necropsy were placed in 10% phosphate-buffered formalin for 24 hours. After fixation, the fragments were dehydrated, diaphanized, embedded in paraffin, cut on a microtome to a thickness of 3.0µm and stained with hematoxylin and eosin (LUNA, 1968).

4.7. Statistical analysis

To evaluate the variables studied, a repeated measures analysis of variance was carried out, with a treatment factor with two levels between the animals (G-1 and G-2) and a time factor with 7 levels (M0, M1, M2, M3, M4, M5 and M6) within the groups.

Tukey's test (P < 0.05) was applied when the main factors and interactions were found to be significant. For two independent samples, a Student's t-test was used with a 5% significance level (VIEIRA, 1998).

---

9 Reflotron, Roche Diagnostic Systems
10 Shimadzu CS 9301 - Tokyo, Japan.
11 Sigma - Saint Louis, USA.

5. RESULTS

5.1. clinical manifestations

Based on the data obtained, it can be seen that the intoxication induction model used was 100% efficient, since all the experimentally intoxicated animals (G-2) showed clinical signs of intoxication and as they were not treated, they died. The total dose of copper given to the sheep until the onset of the hemolytic crisis is described in Table 1.

Table 1 - Total dose of copper sulphate pentahydrate given (g) to sheep in group G-2 and total period of intoxication.

Animals	Total period of intoxication (weeks)	Total dose of copper fed to the animals (g)
2-A	31	147,44
2-B	26	115,18
2-C	33	131,63

The first clinical signs were seen 24 hours before the hemolytic crisis. At this time, the sheep showed signs of inappetence, especially when concentrated feed was offered to the animals, and apathy characterized by sternal decubitus and by not reacting to environmental stimuli, such as food being placed in the feeders. In addition, the animals had slightly pale mucous membranes and no macroscopic hemoglobinuria. At the time of the hemolytic crisis (M4), macroscopic hemoglobinuria could be seen, marked by the brownish color of the urine and yellowish and/or chocolatey eye mucous membranes. There was marked apathy (Figure 1) and the sheep were anorexic. Physical examination revealed tachycardia, tachypnea, mild hypothermia (37.8°C), a capillary refill time of 2-3 seconds, rumen atony, oliguria or anuria. At M5 and M6, the sheep showed prostration, dehydration, tachycardia, tachypnea, CPT greater than 3 seconds, blackish and soft feces (Figure 2), sialorrhea (Figure 3), muscle tremors, bruxism, severe hypothermia (35.6°C), rumen atony, anuria or oliguria, ataxia and uremic halitosis. Lung auscultation at this time revealed the presence of crackles. The survival of the animals after the hemolytic crisis was between 2 and 5 days.

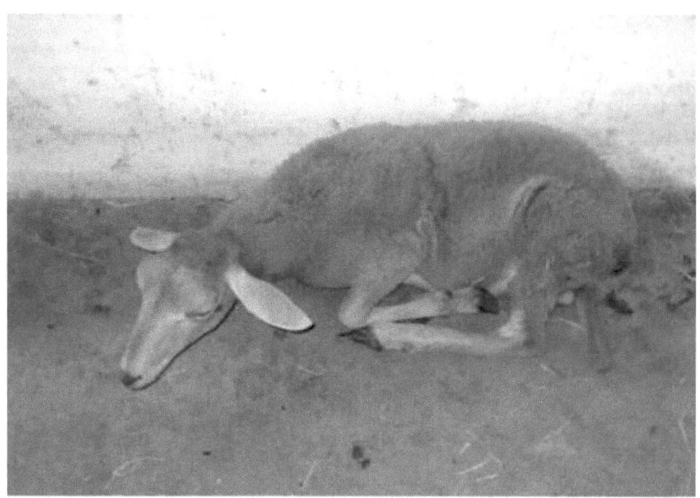

Figura 1 - Apathy in sheep with chronic experimental copper poisoning on the day of the hemolytic crisis.

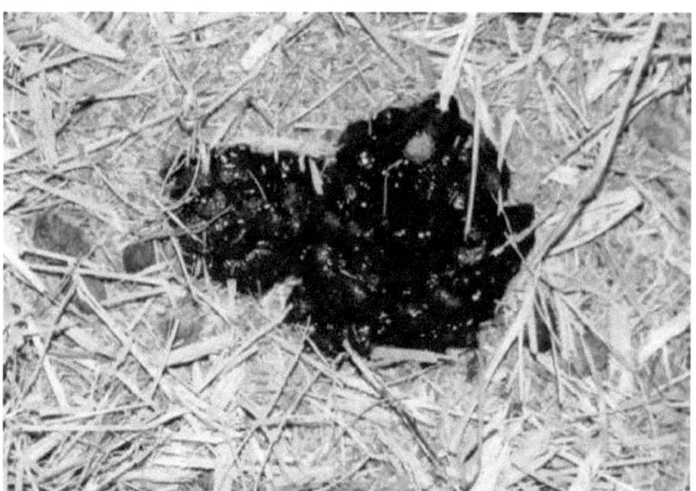

Figura 2 - Blackened and soft feces of sheep with chronic experimental copper intoxication, 48 hours after the hemolytic crisis.

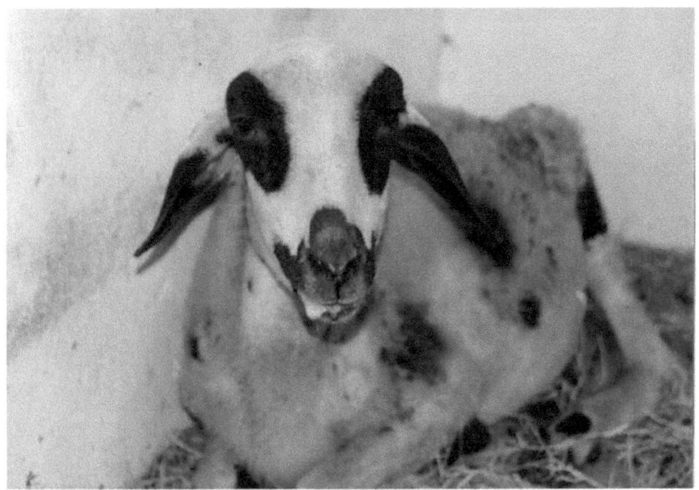

Figura 3 - Prostration and sialorrhea in sheep with chronic experimental copper intoxication, 48 hours after the hemolytic crisis.

5.2. HEMOGRAM

The blood count as well as the leukogram varied within the limits established for the species throughout the pre-hemolytic period (M0 - M3). Considerable changes were only found after the onset of the hemolytic crisis. Table 2 and Figure 4 show the average number of red blood cells in sheep in groups G-1 and G-2.

The number of red blood cells was within the normal range for the species ($9{-}15 \times 10^6/\mu L$, PUGH, 2005) showing that in the intoxication model there were no changes in the red blood cell count before the hemolytic phase of intoxication (M0 - M3). After the onset of the hemolytic crisis (M4 - M6), erythrocyte values declined considerably (P<0.05).

The hematocrit values followed the red blood cell count values, as shown in Table 3.

Table 2 - Mean values and standard deviations of the red blood cell count ($\times 10^6/\mu l$) of sheep in the control group (G-1) and those experimentally intoxicated by copper (G-2), before (M0 - M3), during (M4) and after the hemolytic crisis (M5 and M6).

Groups	MOMENTS						
	M0	M1	M2	M3	M4	M5	M6
G-1	$10{,}0 \pm 0^{Aa}$	$9{,}3 \pm 0{,}6^{Aa}$	$10{,}3 \pm 1{,}6^{Aa}$	$9{,}3 \pm 1{,}5^{Aa}$	$9{,}7 \pm 1{,}5^{Aa}$	$9{,}0 \pm 1{,}0^{Aa}$	$9{,}3 \pm 0{,}6^{Aa}$
G-2	$10{,}3 \pm 0{,}6^{Aa}$	$8{,}7 \pm 0{,}6^{Aa}$	$8{,}7 \pm 1{,}5^{Aa}$	$8{,}3 \pm 1{,}5^{Aa}$	$6{,}0 \pm 1{,}0^{Bb}$	$4{,}7 \pm 2{,}1^{Bb}$	$3{,}3 \pm 1{,}5^{Cb}$

Note: Different capital letters in the same row indicate significant differences (P<0.05) between the moments.

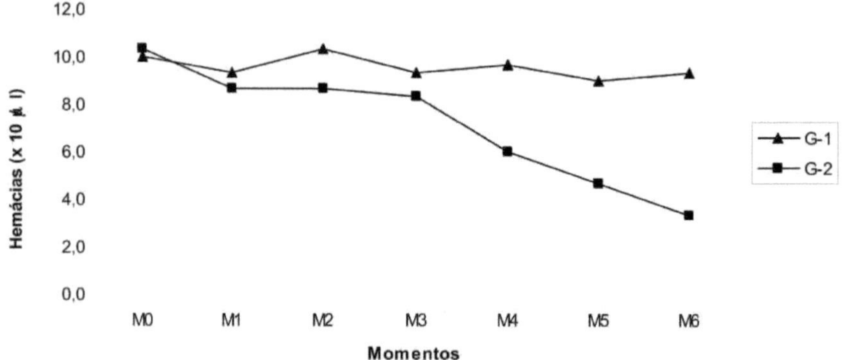

Figure 4 - Graphical representation of the average red blood cell values ($\times 10^6$ /μl) of sheep in the control group (G-1) and those experimentally poisoned by copper (G-2), before (M0 - M3), during (M4) and after the hemolytic crisis (M5 and M6).

Hematocrit values remained within the normal range until the onset of the hemolytic crisis. From 24 hours after the onset of the hemolytic crisis (M5 and M6), these values dropped significantly (P<0.05). The behavior of this component as a function of the time of intoxication is shown in Figure 5.

Table 3 - Mean values and standard deviations of hematocrit (%) of sheep in the control group (G-1) and those experimentally poisoned by copper (G-2), before (M0 - M3), during (M4) and after the hemolytic crisis (M5 and M6).

Groups	Moments						
	M0	M1	M2	M3	M4	M5	M6
G-1	32,7 ±0,6[Aa]	35,0± 1,7[Aa]	34,3± 2,1[Aa]	37,3± 2,5[Aa]	34,3± 4,9[Aa]	36,3± 2,3[Aa]	33,7± 1,2[Aa]
G-2	31,7± 0,6[Aa]	32,6± 2,1[Aa]	31,3± 2,1[Aa]	31,7± 3,1[Aa]	27,3± 6,6[Bb]	18,0± 3,6[Cb]	15,7± 3,1[Cb]

Note: Different capital letters in the same row indicate significant differences (P<0.05) between the moments. Distinct lower-case letters in the columns indicate significant differences (P<0.05) between the groups.

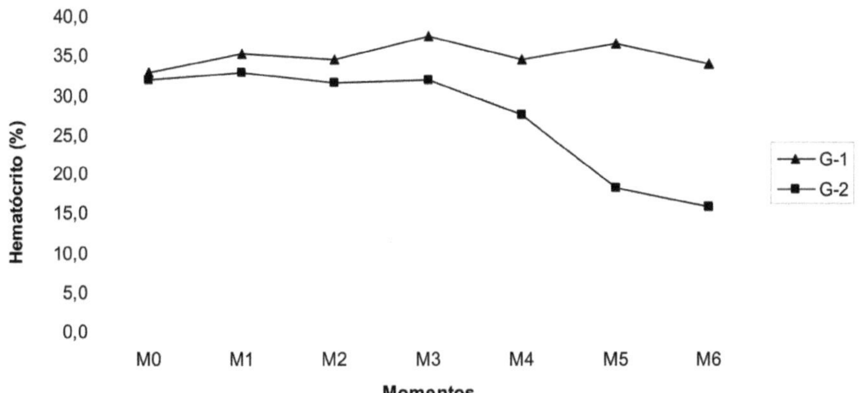

Figure 5 - Graphical representation of the average hematocrit values (%) of sheep in the control group (G-1) and those experimentally poisoned by copper (G-2), before (M0 - M3), during (M4) and after the hemolytic crisis (M5 and M6).

The hemoglobin levels remained unchanged between the sheep in groups G-1 and G-2 at times M0, M1, M2 and M3, varying within the values established for the species (10 - 15.4 g/dL, PUGH, 2005). From M4 onwards, which represents the onset of the hemolytic crisis, there was a significant reduction (P<0.05) in the hemoglobin levels of the G-2 animals, when compared to G-1 and the previous moments (Table 4 and Figure 6).

Table 4 - Mean values and standard deviations of hemoglobin (g/dL) of sheep in the control group (G-1) and those experimentally poisoned by copper (G-2), before (M0 - M3), during (M4) and after the hemolytic crisis (M5 and M6).

Groups	Moments						
	M0	M1	M2	M3	M4	M5	M6
G-1	$10,5\pm 0,4^{Aa}$	$10,0\pm 3,4^{Aa}$	$10,3\pm 3,4^{Aa}$	$9,3\pm 3,68^{Aa}$	$8,9\pm 1,4^{Aa}$	$8,6\pm 0,95^{Aa}$	$8,6\pm 0,7^{Aa}$
G-2	$10,0\pm 0,3^{Aa}$	$9,2\pm 3,0^{Aa}$	$8,7\pm 1,8^{Aa}$	$8,7\pm 2,8^{Aa}$	$5,8\pm 1,6^{Bb}$	$4,2\pm 1,0^{Bb}$	$3,8\pm 1,2^{Bb}$

Note: Different capital letters in the same row indicate significant differences (P<0.05) between the moments. Distinct lower-case letters in the columns indicate significant differences (P<0.05) between the groups.

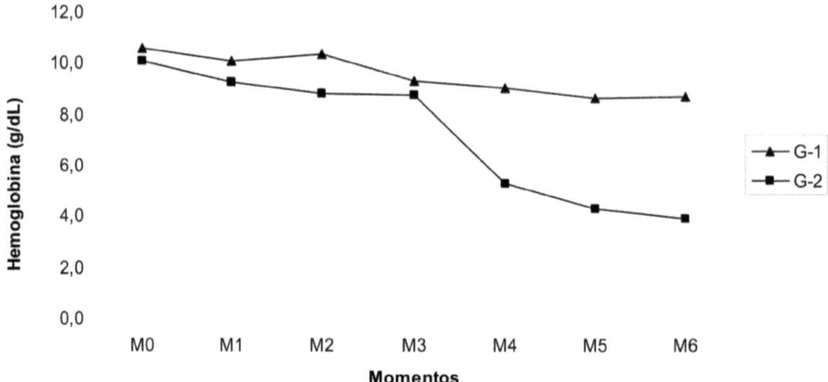

Figure 6 - Graphical representation of the average hemoglobin values (g/dL) of sheep in the control group (G-1) and those experimentally poisoned by copper (G-2), before (M0 - M3), during (M4) and after the hemolytic crisis (M5 and M6).

Based on the red blood cell, hematocrit and hemoglobin values, the hematimetric indices were calculated (Tables 5 and 6). Figure 7 shows the behavior of the mean corpuscular volume (MCV) of erythrocytes as a function of time, while Figure 8 shows the kinetics of the mean corpuscular hemoglobin (MCHC) values. The values considered normal are 28 - 40 fL for MCV and 31-34 g/dL for MCHC, according to PUGH (2005).

Until M3, the sheep in groups G-1 and G-2 had normocytic and normochromic red blood cells. When the hemolytic process began (M4), the sheep in group G-2 began to show a macrocytic normochromic anemia that lasted two days, while the red blood cells of the sheep in group G-1 remained normocytic and normochromic.

Table 5 - Mean values and standard deviations of the mean corpuscular volume (fL) of sheep in the control group (G-1) and those experimentally poisoned by copper (G-2), before (M0 - M3), during (M4) and after the hemolytic crisis (M5 and M6).

Groups	Moments						
	M0	M1	M2	M3	M4	M5	M6
G-1	$31,9 \pm 0,9^{Aa}$	$35,9 \pm 0,9^{Aa}$	$32,1 \pm 3,9^{Aa}$	$38,1 \pm 3,5^{Aa}$	$33,7 \pm 2,0^{Aa}$	$37,4 \pm 2,0^{Aa}$	$33,7 \pm 0,4^{Aa}$
G-2	$29,1 \pm 2,2^{Aa}$	$35,9 \pm 3,2^{Aa}$	$33,5 \pm 0,7^{Aa}$	$35,8 \pm 6,6^{Aa}$	$44,1 \pm 13,9^{Bb}$	$45,3 \pm 15,5^{Bb}$	$36,9 \pm 9,3^{Aa}$

Note: Different capital letters in the same row indicate significant differences (P<0.05) between the moments. Distinct lower-case letters in the columns indicate significant differences (P<0.05) between the groups.

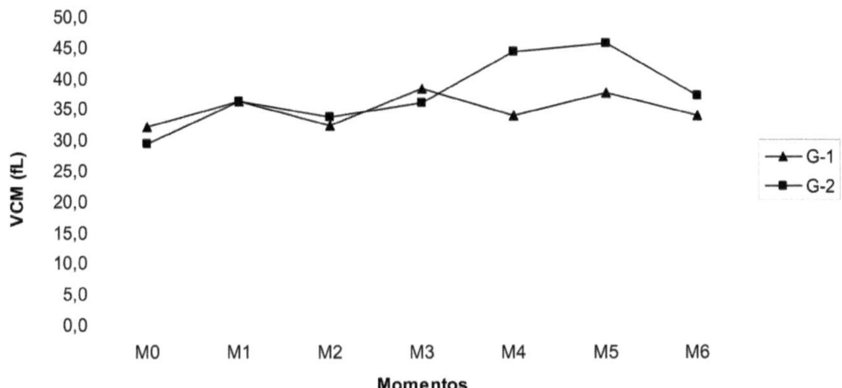

Figure 7 - Graphical representation of the mean corpuscular volume values (fL) of sheep in the control group (G-1) and those experimentally poisoned by copper (G- 2), before (MO - M3), during (M4) and after the hemolytic crisis (M5 and M6).

Table 6 - Mean values and standard deviations of the mean corpuscular hemoglobin concentration (g/dL) of sheep in the control group (G-1) and those experimentally poisoned by copper (G-2), before (MO - M3), during (M4) and after the hemolytic crisis (M5 and M6).

Groups	Moments						
	M0	**M1**	**M2**	**M3**	**M4**	**M5**	**M6**
G-1	$32,3 \pm 1,6^{Aa}$	$28,3 \pm 8,0^{Aa}$	$29,9 \pm 9,5^{Aa}$	$24,5 \pm 7,8^{Aa}$	$26,1 \pm 0,4^{Aa}$	$23,5 \pm 1,6^{Aa}$	$25,6 \pm 1,8^{Aa}$
G-2	$31,6 \pm 0,6^{Aa}$	$28,2 \pm 9,7^{Aa}$	$27,7 \pm 3,9^{Aa}$	$27,5 \pm 9,4^{Aa}$	$25,23 \pm 10,7^{Aa}$	$25,2 \pm 2,5^{Aa}$	$26,1 \pm 7,4^{Aa}$

Note: Different capital letters in the same row indicate significant differences (P<0.05) between the moments. Distinct lower-case letters in the columns indicate significant differences (P<0.05) between the groups.

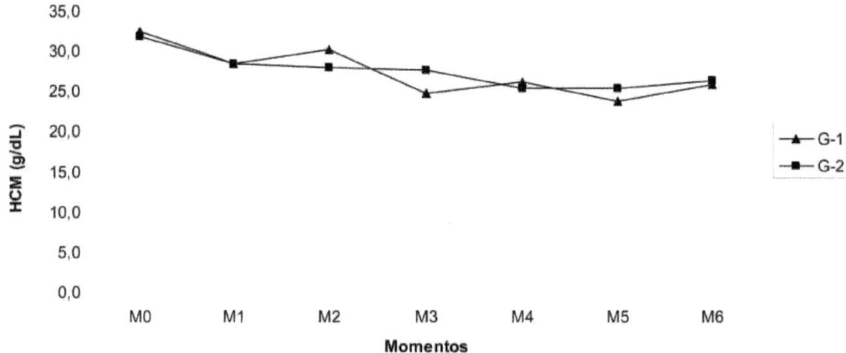

Figure 8 - Graphical representation of the average values of the mean corpuscular hemoglobin concentration (g/dL) of sheep in the control group (G-1) and those experimentally poisoned by copper (G-2), before (M0 - M3), during (M4) and after the hemolytic crisis (M5 and M6).

5.3. Scanning Electron Microscopy

During the pre-hemolytic phase of copper intoxication (M0 - M3), 85% of the red blood cells visualized by scanning electron microscopy had a normal pattern, also known as discoid (Figure 9). However, at moments M2 and M3 of this phase, the morphological pattern of the erythrocytes began to change and other forms of red blood cells, such as macrocytes (Figure 10A and 10B), kinizocytes (Figure 10C) and dacryocytes (Figure 10D) began to be seen in greater proportions. When the hemolytic crisis was triggered, there were marked and persistent changes in the morphology of the red blood cells of the sheep in group G-2 (Figures 11 and 12).

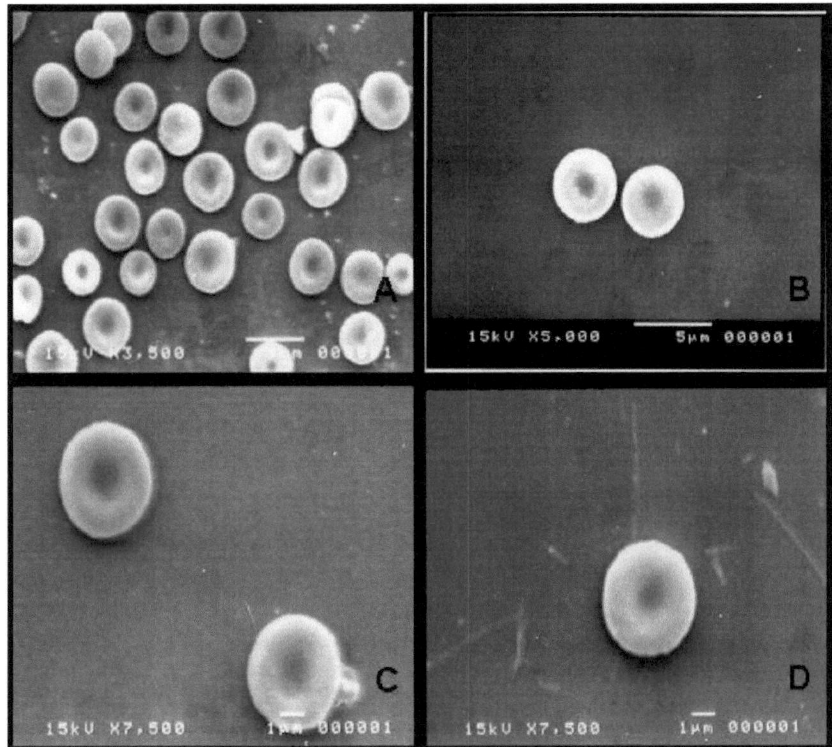

Figure 9 - Electromicrograph of sheep red blood cells during the pre-hemolytic phase (M0 - M3) of cumulative copper intoxication. A, B, C and D - Normal appearance of sheep red blood cells (discocytes) at MO and M1 of cumulative copper intoxication at different magnifications.

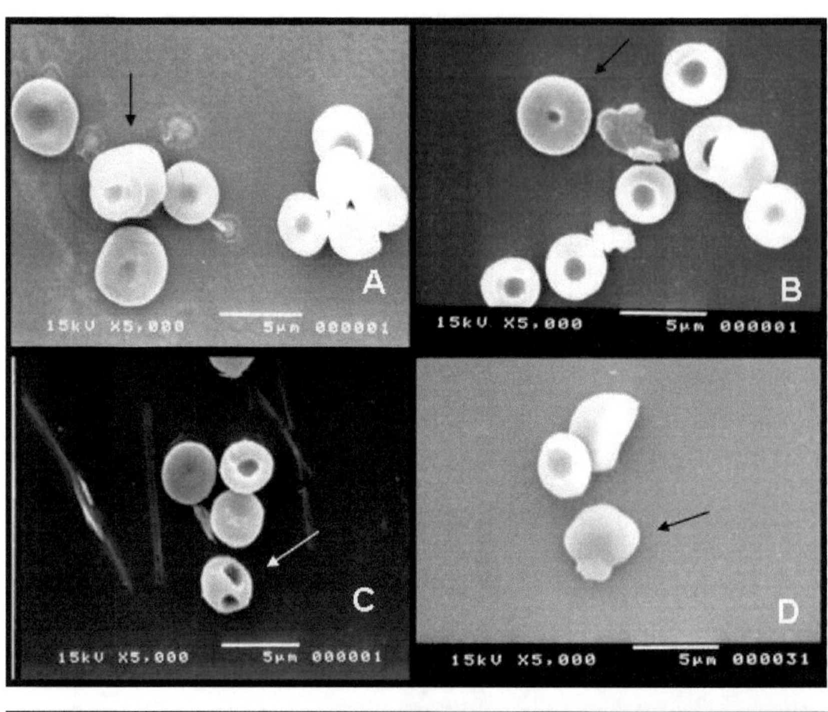

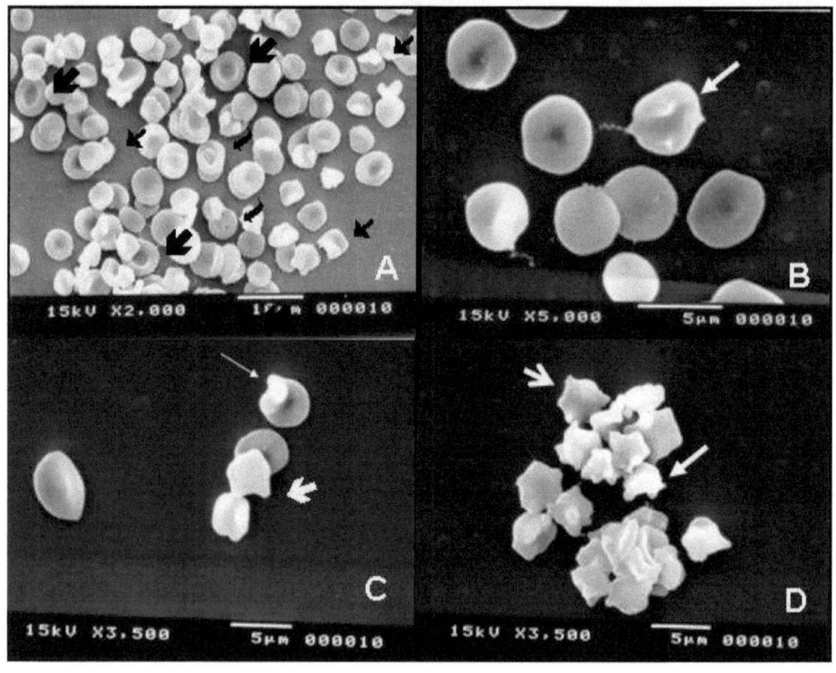

Figure 11 - Electromicrograph of sheep red blood cells during the hemolytic phase (M4 - M6) of cumulative copper intoxication. M4: A - Loss of morphological homogeneity of the red blood cells, which appear in different forms: macrocytes (4^I), acanthocytes ($\square$), and codocytes (K); B - Presence of stomatocytes ($\square$). M5: C - Presence of acanthocytes (K) and Heinz corpuscle ($\square$). M6: D - Marked changes in cell pattern and presence of acanthocytes (D) and Heinz corpuscle ($\square$).

Figure 12 - Electromicrograph of sheep red blood cells during the hemolytic phase (M4 - M6) of cumulative copper intoxication. M6: A - Marked changes in the cellular pattern; B - keratocyte; C - Presence of hemoglobin crystals deposited on the membrane of an erythrocyte; D - Heinz corpuscle.

5.4. Leukometry

As with the red blood cells, there were no changes in the leukocyte count between M0 and M3, as shown in Table 7. The values remained within the normal range for the species (4,000 to 12,000/ μl - PUGH, 2005). From moment M4 onwards, the number of total leukocytes increased, reaching significant values ($P<0.05$) at moments M5 and M6. The behavior of the leukocytes as a function of the time of intoxication is shown in Figure 13.

The leukocytosis seen at times M4, M5 and M6 was due to an increase in segmented neutrophils, this increase being significant ($P<0.05$) at times M5 and M6 (Table 8 and Figure 14). Lymphocytes, on the other hand, remained at the reference values for the species (2,000 to 9,000/ μl - PUGH, 2005), but showed a reduction when compared to the values of group G-1 (Table 9 and Figure 15).

Table 7 - Mean values and standard deviations of total leukocytes ($\times 10^3$/ μL) of sheep in the control group (G-1) and those experimentally poisoned by copper (G-2), before (M0 - M3), during (M4) and after the hemolytic crisis (M5 and M6).

GROUPS	MOMENTS						
	MO	**M1**	**M2**	**M3**	**M4**	**M5**	**M6**
G-1	$10{,}6 \pm 2{,}9^{Aa}$	$7{,}7 \pm 1{,}7^{Aa}$	$8{,}4 \pm 2{,}2^{Aa}$	$7{,}2 \pm 1{,}6^{Aa}$	$8{,}3 \pm 2{,}0^{Aa}$	$8{,}6 \pm 0{,}9^{Aa}$	$9{,}1 \pm 0{,}8^{Aa}$
G-2	$10{,}7 \pm 4{,}7^{Aa}$	$11{,}7 \pm 3{,}9^{Aa}$	$9{,}9 \pm 1{,}2^{Aa}$	$8{,}3 \pm 1{,}3^{Aa}$	$12{,}6 \pm 7{,}2^{Aa}$	$14{,}6 \pm 5{,}3^{Bb}$	$15{,}4 \pm 8{,}3^{Bb}$

Note: Different capital letters in the same row indicate significant differences ($P<0.05$) between the moments. Distinct lower-case letters in the columns indicate significant differences ($P<0.05$) between the groups.

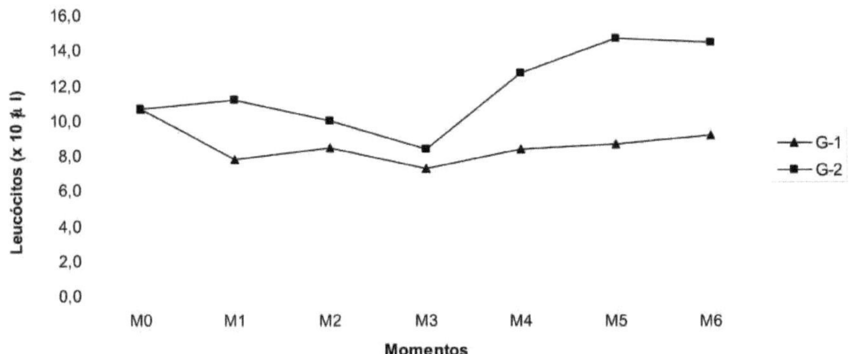

Figure 13 - Graphical representation of the average total leukocyte count (x10^3 / µL) of sheep in the control group (G-1) and those experimentally poisoned by copper (G- 2), before (M0 - M3), during (M4) and after the hemolytic crisis (M5 and M6).

Table 8 - Mean values and standard deviations of segmented neutrophils (x10^3 / µL) of sheep in the control group (G-1) and those experimentally poisoned by copper (G-2), before (M0 - M3), during (M4) and after the hemolytic crisis (M5 and M6).

Groups	Moments						
	M0	M1	M2	M3	M4	M5	M6
G-1	$3,4 \pm 1,1^{Aa}$	$2,1 \pm 0,5^{Aa}$	$2,4 \pm 0,5^{Aa}$	$1,6 \pm 0,3^{Aa}$	$2,7 \pm 0,3^{Aa}$	$2,6 \pm 0,7^{Aa}$	$2,8 \pm 0,555^{Aa}$
G-2	$4,3 \pm 1,5^{Aa}$	$3,6 \pm 1,6^{Aa}$	$3,6 \pm 0,7^{Aa}$	$3,2 \pm 0,7^{Ab}$	$6,9 \pm 4,6^{Ab}$	$8,6 \pm 5,3^{Bb}$	$10,6 \pm 5,8^{Bb}$

Note: Different capital letters in the same row indicate significant differences (P<0.05) between the moments. Distinct lower-case letters in the columns indicate significant differences (P<0.05) between the groups.

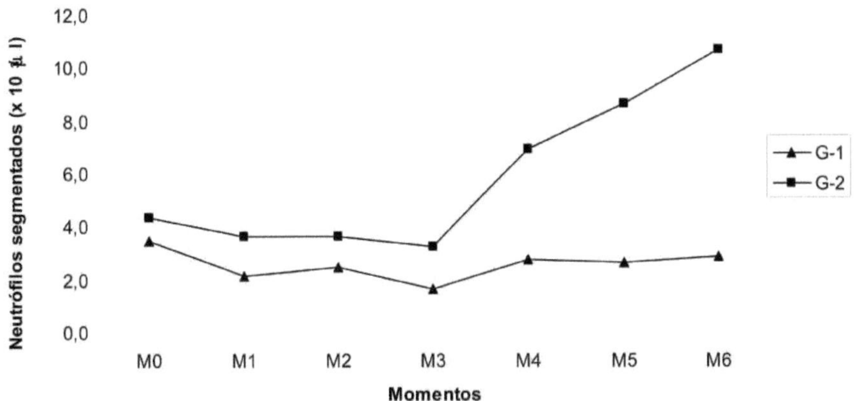

Figure 14 - Graphical representation of the mean values and standard deviations of segmented neutrophils (x10^3 / µL) in sheep from the control group (G-1) and those experimentally intoxicated by copper (G-2), before (M0 - M3), during (M4) and after the hemolytic crisis (M5 and M6).

Table 9 - Mean values and standard deviations of lymphocytes (x10^3 / µL) of sheep in the control group (G-1) and those experimentally intoxicated by copper (G-2), before (M0 - M3), during (M4) and after the hemolytic crisis (M5 and M6).

Groups	Moments						
	M0	M1	M2	M3	M4	M5	M6
G-1	6,8 ± 3,0[Aa]	5,5 ± 1,9[Aa]	5,7 ± 1,9[Aa]	5,4 ± 1,7[Aa]	5,4 ± 1,9[Aa]	5,8 ± 1,6[Aa]	6,0 ± 1,3[Aa]
G-2	5,6 ± 3,3[Aa]	5,9 ± 2,2[Aa]	5,7 ± 0,8[Aa]	4,7 ± 0,9[Aa]	4,6 ± 1,3[Aa]	5,4 ± 1,5[Aa]	4,4 ± 2,1[Aa]

Note: Different capital letters in the same row indicate significant differences (P<0.05) between the moments. Distinct lower-case letters in the columns indicate significant differences (P<0.05) between the groups.

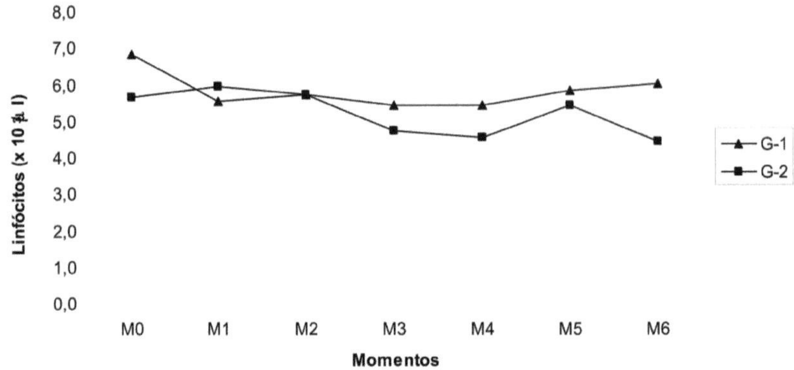

Figure 15 - Graphical representation of the average lymphocyte values ($x10^3$ / µL) of sheep in the control group (G-1) and those experimentally intoxicated by copper (G-2), before (M0 - M3), during (M4) and after the hemolytic crisis (M5 and M6).

5.5. Biochemical analysis of blood serum

The activities of AST, GGT and CK are shown in Tables 10, 11 and 12. The AST values showed that the activity of this enzyme remained within the values established for the species at all times in the G-1 animals. In relation to G-2, it can be seen that the serum activity of this enzyme increased significantly from M2 onwards, although in M3 its activity was more marked. In M4, the activity of this enzyme reached higher values, but the highest activity was detected in M6. The kinetics of this enzyme are shown in Figure 16.

Table 10 - Mean serum activities and standard deviations of the enzyme aspartate aminotransferase (U/L) of sheep in the control group (G-1) and those experimentally intoxicated by copper (G-2), before (M0 - M3), during (M4) and after the hemolytic crisis (M5 and M6) _________________ '.

Groups	Moments						
	M0	M1	M2	M3	M4	M5	M6
G-1	86 ± 15^{Aa}	86 ± 15^{Aa}	103 ± 29^{Aa}	96 ± 13^{Aa}	70 ± 4^{Aa}	96 ± 23^{Aa}	130 ± 45^{Aa}
G-2	$139 \pm 22A^{b}$	$137 \pm 14A^{b}$	$177 \pm 20B^{b}$	388 ± 76^{cb}	567 ± 134^{cb}	440 ± 65^{cb}	$1030 \pm 552B^{b}$

Note: Different capital letters in the same row indicate significant differences (P<0.05) between the moments. Distinct lower-case letters in the columns indicate significant differences (P<0.05) between the groups.

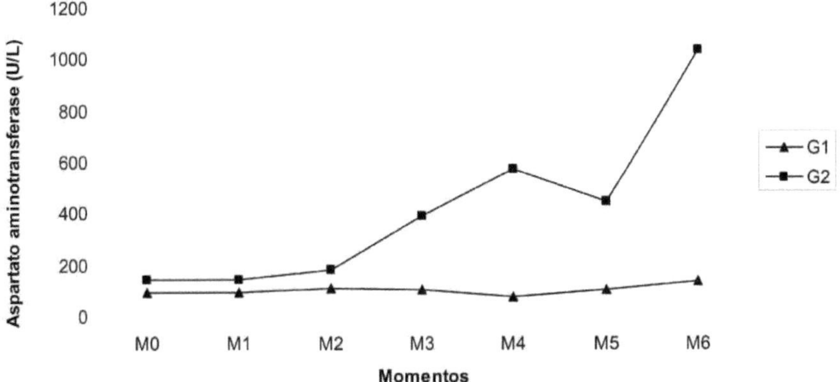

Figure 16 - Graphical representation of the average serum activities of the enzyme aspartate aminotransferase (U/L) of sheep in the control group (G-1) and those experimentally poisoned by copper (G-2), before (M0 - M3), during (M4) and after the hemolytic crisis (M5 and M6).

Table 11 shows the average values of the gamma glutamyltransferase enzyme at different times. The kinetics of this enzyme are shown in Figure 17.

Table 11 - Mean serum activities and standard deviations of the enzyme gamma-glutamyltransferase (U/L) of sheep in the control group (G-1) and those experimentally poisoned by copper (G-2), before (M0 - M3), during (M4) and after the hemolytic crisis (M5 and M6).

Groups	Moments						
	M0	M1	M2	M3	M4	M5	M6
G-1	62 ± 2^{Aa}	60 ± 3^{Aa}	71 ± 23^{Aa}	71 ± 15^{Aa}	57 ± 11^{Aa}	66 ± 15^{Aa}	71 ± 15^{Aa}
G-2	74 ± 10^{Ab}	103 ± 28^{Ab}	175 ± 75^{Bb}	379 ± 156^{Bb}	486 ± 286^{Bb}	302 ± 147^{Bb}	193 ± 71^{Bb}

Note: Different capital letters in the same row indicate significant differences (P<0.05) between the moments. Distinct lower-case letters in the columns indicate significant differences (P<0.05) between the groups.

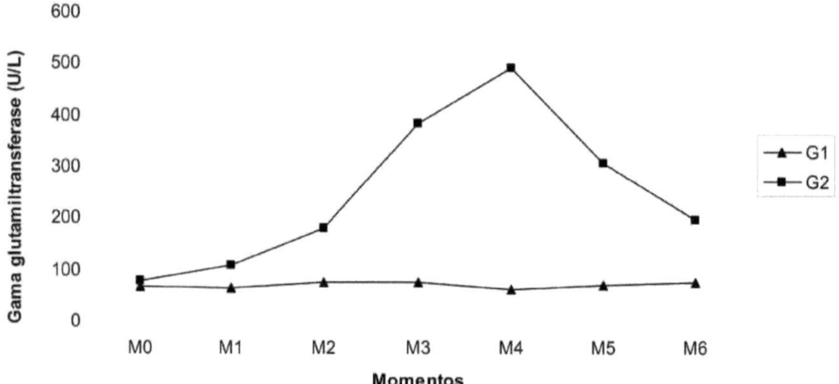

Figure 17 - Graphical representation of the average serum gamma glutamyltransferase levels (U/L) of sheep in the control group (G-1) and those experimentally poisoned by copper (G-2), before (M0 - M3), during (M4) and after the hemolytic crisis (M5 and M6).

Serum GGT activity remained higher than the values established for the species in both G-1 and G-2 sheep. In the G-2 sheep, the enzyme gamma-glutamyltransferase was an excellent indicator of the hemolytic crisis, since it showed increased activity when compared to the G-1 animals, reaching serum levels 40% higher than at baseline (M0) at M2. Subsequently, serum GGT activity increased significantly until M4. After the onset of the hemolytic crisis, serum GGT activity decreased, but remained above the values established for the species.

Serum CK activity (Table 12) showed significant changes only at times M4 to M6 in the G-2 sheep. No increase in serum CK activity was observed in the G-1 sheep. The kinetics of the creatine kinase enzyme are shown in Figure 18.

Table 12 - Mean serum activities and standard deviations of the creatine kinase enzyme (U/L) of sheep in the control group (G-1) and those experimentally poisoned by copper (G-2), before (M0 - M3), during (M4) and after the hemolytic crisis (M5 and M6).

				Moments			
Groups	**MO**	**M1**	**M2**	**M3**	**M4**	**M5**	**M6**
G-1	51 ± 13^{Aa}	62 ± 24^{Aa}	110 ± 50^{Aa}	39 ± 4^{Aa}	31 ± 3^{Ba}	54 ± 17^{Aa}	95 ± 44^{Aa}
G-2	54 ± 4^{Aa}	168 ± 172^{Aa}	43 ± 12^{Aa}	35 ± 6^{Ba}	89 ± 65^{Ab}	436 ± 219^{Cb}	840 ± 385^{Cb}

Note: Different capital letters in the same row indicate significant differences (P<0.05) between the moments. Distinct lower-case letters in the columns indicate significant differences (P<0.05) between times.

grupos.

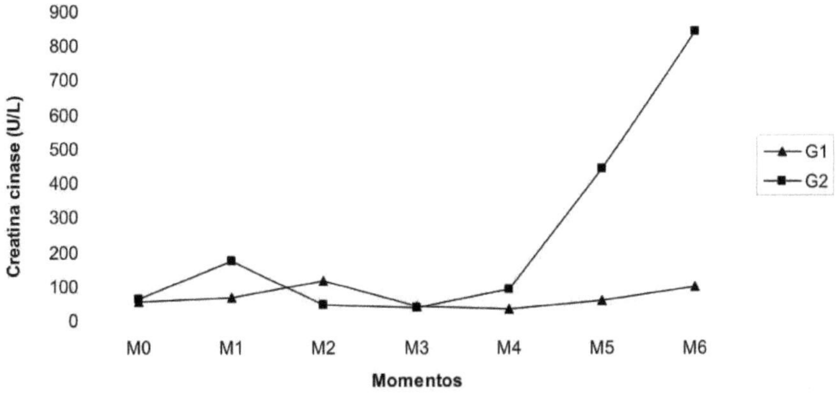

Figure 18 - Graphical representation of the average serum creatine kinase activities (U/L) of sheep in the control group (G-1) and those experimentally poisoned by copper (G-2), before (M0 - M3), during (M4) and after the hemolytic crisis (M5 and M6).

5.6. Serum Proteinogram

Acrylamide gel electrophoresis containing sodium dodecyl sulfate (SDS-PAGE) allowed the identification of different protein fractions with molecular weights ranging from 22,000 to 260,000 daltons (Da) in six sheep. Among the protein fractions identified (Table 13), it was clear that the protein with a molecular weight of 122,000 Da (ceruloplasmin) maintained its levels below baseline values throughout the course of intoxication, increasing only at the M5 moment of cumulative copper intoxication. On the other hand, proteins with a molecular weight of 83,000 Da (transferrin), 35,000 Da and 27,000 Da (light chain IgG) increased by 326, 128 and 22% respectively in the 15 days prior to the hemolytic crisis (M2). The percentage variation of these proteins is described in Table 14, and their kinetics are shown in Figures 20, 21, 22 and 23.

Table 13 - Mean values and standard deviations of serum protein concentrations, obtained by sodium dodecyl sulphate-acrylamide gel electrophoresis (SDS-PAGE) of sheep from the control group (G-1) and those experimentally intoxicated by copper (G-2), before (M0 - M3), during (M4) and after the hemolytic crisis (M5 and M6).

Protein (PM) and	MOMENTS													
	M0		M1		M2		M3		M4		M5		M6	
	Average	DP	Average	DP	Average	DP	Average	DP	Average	DP	Average	DP	Average	DP

Total serum protein (g/dL)								
G-1	6,1	0,4 5,9	0,7 5,9	0,3 5,6	0,4 5,9	1,0 6,0	1,1 7,5	0,6
G-2	6,3	0,2 5,8	0,2 6,0	0,3 5,8	0,4 5,9	0,1 5,7	0,2 5,9	0,6
α-lipoprotein (PM 232,000; mg/dL)								
G-1	3,9	0,6 2,6	0,9 3,6	4,5 8,2	5,0 5,8	2,5 5,9	2,9 8,4	6,7
G-2	7,2	5,9 4,4	3,8 2,8	2,6 7,5	2,3 6,5	3,3 2,3	1,1 5,7	7,0
Ceruloplasmin (PM 122,000; mg/dL)								
G-1	20,1	6,4 16,0	3,8 24,6	11,0 17,3	5,0 15,3	7,1 23,0	14,8 19,4	9,1
G-2	28,8	11,3 21,0	14,8 19,3	7,9 26,5	4,2 28,0	16,4 39,4	23,3 22,7	18,5
PM 109,000 (mg/dL)								
G-1	23,8	12,7 19,3	5,8 22,6	6,7 18,7	7,3 17,6	6,6 15,0	11,8 30,6	10,9
G-2	26,1	12,7 24,6	5,0 22,6	12,6 18,6	8,6 32,9	11,9 28,9	17,6 26,6	12,2
C-reactive protein (PM 102,000; mg/dL)								
G-1	5,2	0,1 7,3	1,8 7,4	0,9 10,0	3,8 6,1	3,8 6,5	2,5 7,4	1,2
G-2	9,0	2,4 8,4	1,7 9,6	0,8 6,7	1,7 9,6	1,2 9,1	2,2 8,9	2,2
Transferrin (PM 83,000; mg/dL)								
G-1	235	48 216	67 217	28 220	72 285	85 300	48 553	191
G-2	204	149 318	117 460	203 264	153 359	194 228	55 242	200
Albumin (PM 65,000; g/dL)								
G-	4,4	0,6 4,4	0,6 4,0	0,1 3,8	0,8 3,8	0,9 3,8	1,3 4,6	1,3
G^ntinuation	4,2	0,3 3,7	0,6 3,7	0,6 3,6	0,9 3,5	0,3 3,6	0,1 3,9	0,8
IgG heavy chain (PM 55,000; mg/dL)								
G-1	939	426 661	150 870	118 836	209 956	15 852	97 1201	306
G-2	934	69 1016	283 1063	252 1076	366 1117	173 1048	280 1035	250
PM 35,000 (mg/dL)								
G-1	10,5	6,6 4,6	2,5 10,5	11,5 5,9	8,4 4,2	2,0 9,1	3,8 53,5	44,3
G-2	5,4	3,1 7,5	6,8 23,2	18,2 11,9	15,9 17,5	17,6 5,9	3,6 9,2	3,7
IgG light chain (PM 27,000; mg/dL)								
G-1	238	230 261	147 290	51 291	92 318	23 301	45 441	184
G-2	297	45 302	288 361	185 174	153 444	183 380	178 394	194
PM 25,000 (mg/dL)								
G-1	89,8	20,8 105,5	28,0 117,1	20,4 104,2	19,0 111,6	27,4 124,5	28,1 149,2	44,8
G-2	137,6	26,1 105,7	21,3 127,6	13,3 90,3	20,3 119,0	18,1 113,4	24,4 132,9	25,7

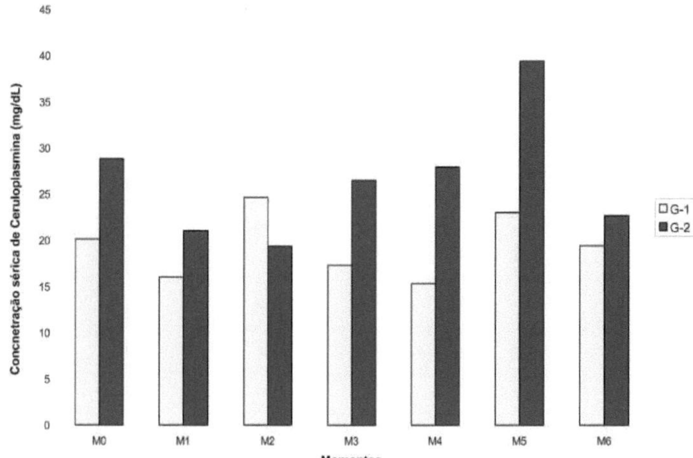

FIGURA 19 - Graphical representation of the serum concentration of Ceruloplasmin (mg/dL) of sheep in the control group (G-1) and those experimentally poisoned by copper (G-2), before (M0 - M3), during (M4) and after the hemolytic crisis (M5 and M6).

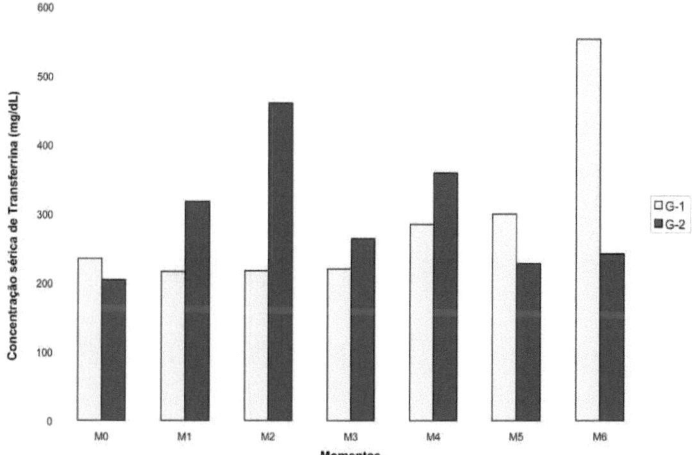

FIGURA 20 - Graphical representation of the serum transferrin concentration (mg/dL) of sheep in the control group (G-1) and those experimentally poisoned by copper (G-2), before (M0 - M3), during (M4) and after the hemolytic crisis (M5 and M6).

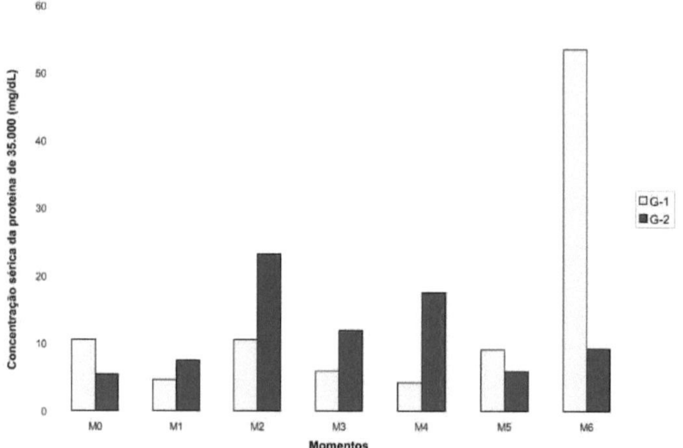

FIGURA 21 - Graphical representation of the serum concentration of the 35,000 Da protein (mg/dL) of sheep in the control group (G-1) and those experimentally poisoned by copper (G-2), before (M0 - M3), during (M4) and after the hemolytic crisis (M5 and M6).

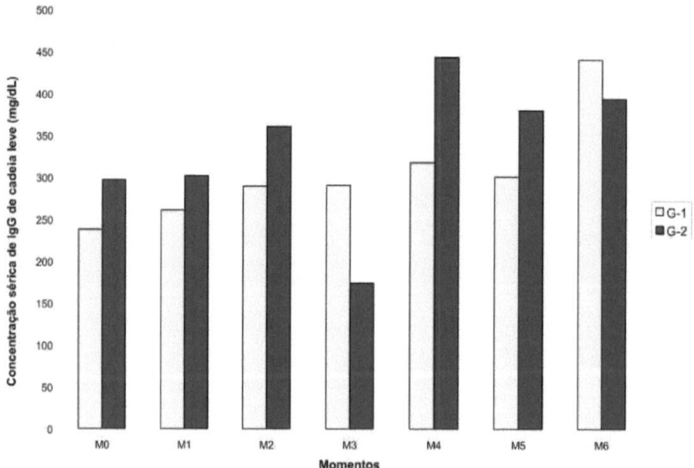

FIGURA 22 - Graphical representation of the serum light chain IgG concentration (mg/dL) of sheep in the control group (G-1) and those experimentally poisoned by copper (G-2), before (M0 - M3), during (M4) and after the hemolytic crisis (M5 and M6).

Table 14 - Variation (%) of serum protein concentrations compared to baseline concentrations in sheep experimentally subjected to cumulative copper intoxication (G-2).

Protein (PM)	Moments

34

	M1	M2	M3	M4	M5	M6
Ceruloplasmin	-27	-33	-8	-3	37	-21
Transferrin	56	126	30	76	12	19
PM 35,000	38	328	120	223	8	70
IgG light chain	2	22	-42	49	28	33

5.7. Serum Copper Levels

Serum copper levels remained within normal limits for the species (9.13 to 25.2 µmol/L - PUGH, 2005) throughout the pre-hemolytic phase, corresponding to moments M0 to M3; however, the animals in group G-2, which received copper sulphate, maintained significantly higher serum copper levels (P<0.05) when compared to the control group (Table 15).

The data presented in Table 09 shows that when the onset of the hemolytic crisis was detected, serum copper levels increased significantly

(P<0.05) and remained high for another 72 hours. The kinetics of this microelement are

shown in Figure 24.

Table 15 - Mean values and standard deviations of serum copper levels (µmol/L) of sheep in the control group (G-1) and those experimentally intoxicated by copper (G-2), before (M0 - M3), during (M4) and after the hemolytic crisis (M5 and M6).

GROUPS	MOMENTS						
	MO	M1	M2	M3	M4	M5	M6
G-1	$11,5 \pm 0,4^{Aa}$	$8,3 \pm 1,7^{Aa}$	$8,7 \pm 1,7^{Aa}$	$9,9 \pm 2,7^{Aa}$	$8,6 \pm 2,7^{Aa}$	$10,9 \pm 5,6^{Aa}$	$8,8 \pm 2,3^{Aa}$
G-2	$14,3 \pm 0,9^{Aa}$	$19,3 \pm 12,4^{Ab}$	$15,6 \pm 4,0^{Ab}$	$17,6 \pm 5,5^{Ab}$	$136,8 \pm 96,0^{Bb}$	$66,2 \pm 35,8^{Cb}$	$48,0 \pm 26,6^{Cb}$

Note: Different capital letters in the same row indicate significant differences (P<0.05) between the moments. Distinct lower-case letters in the columns indicate significant differences (P<0.05) between the groups.

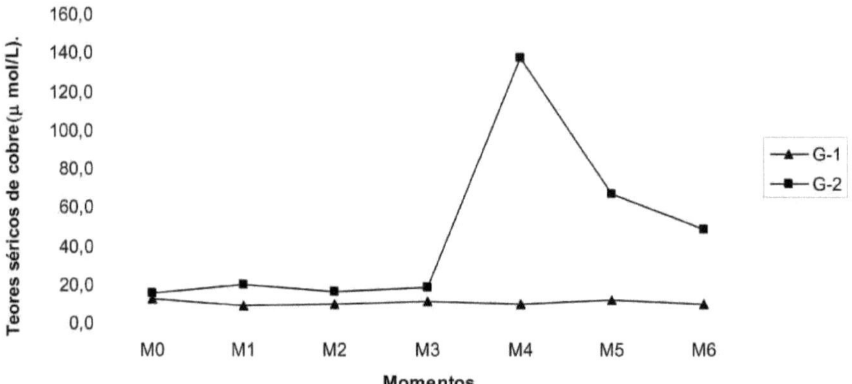

Figure 23 - Graphical representation of the mean values of serum copper levels (µmol/L) in sheep from the control group (G-1) and those experimentally intoxicated by copper (G-2), before (M0 - M3), during (M4) and after the hemolytic crisis (M5 and M6).

5.8. NECROPSY FINDINGS

5.8.1.   Macroscopic findings

The necropsy of the sheep in group G-2 revealed alterations such as: pale or yellowish eye and oral mucous membranes, diffuse jaundice, pulmonary edema, an enlarged, yellowish liver with rounded edges. The spleens of the intoxicated animals were congested and larger than those of the sheep in the control group, the kidneys were blackened after removal of the renal capsule, and the urinary bladders showed amber-colored urine due to hemoglobinuria resulting from hemolytic anemia. The main necropsy findings are shown in Figures 24 to 33. No noteworthy changes were found in the sheep in the control group.

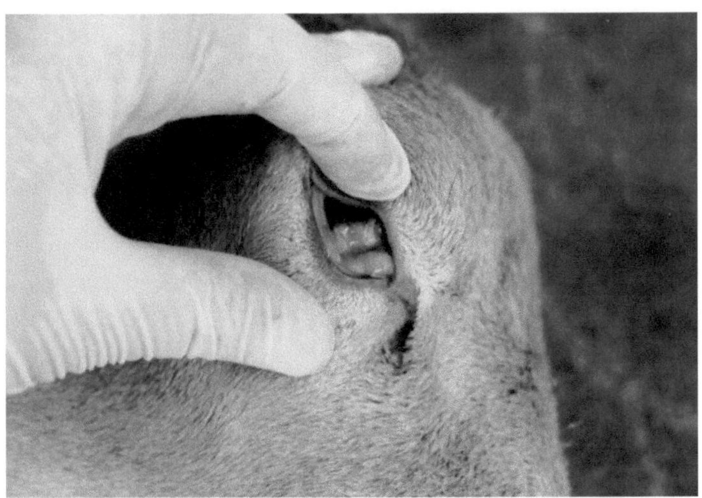

Figure 24 - Icteric ocular mucosa of sheep with chronic experimental copper poisoning.

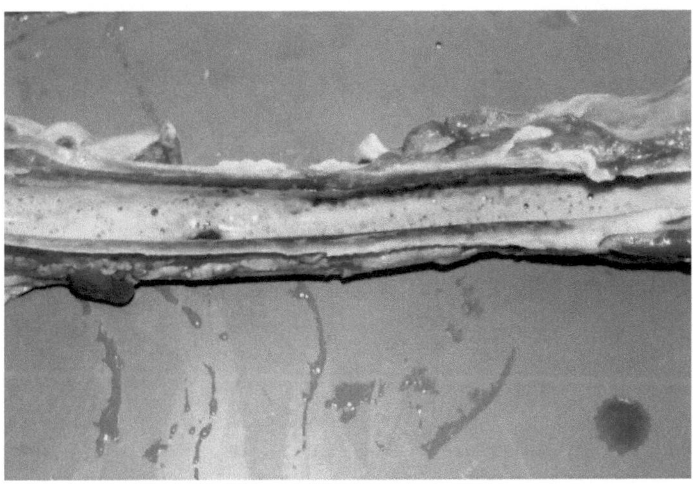

Figure 25 - Foamy liquid in the trachea of sheep with chronic experimental copper poisoning.

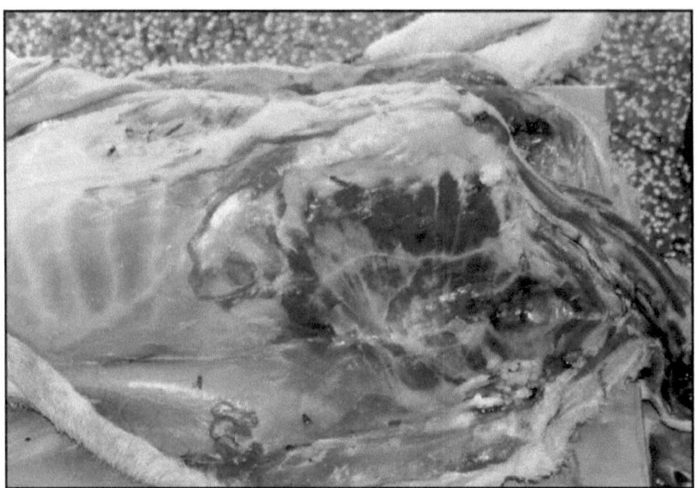

Figure 26 - Icteric subcutaneous, adipose and muscular tissues of sheep with chronic experimental copper poisoning.

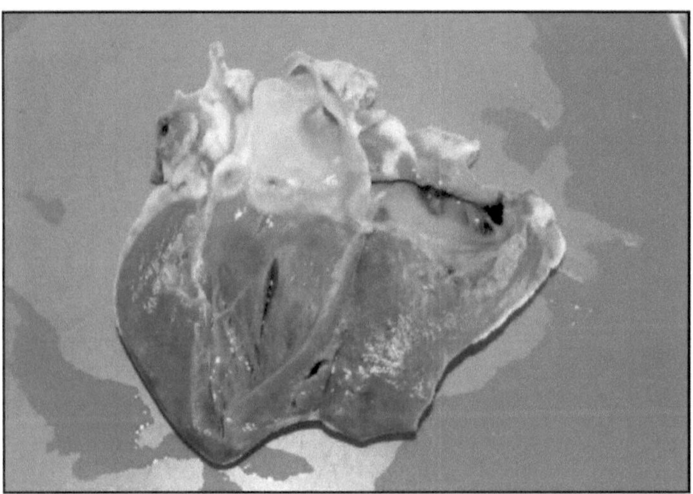

Figure 27 - Icteric large vessels of the cardiac base in sheep with chronic experimental copper poisoning.

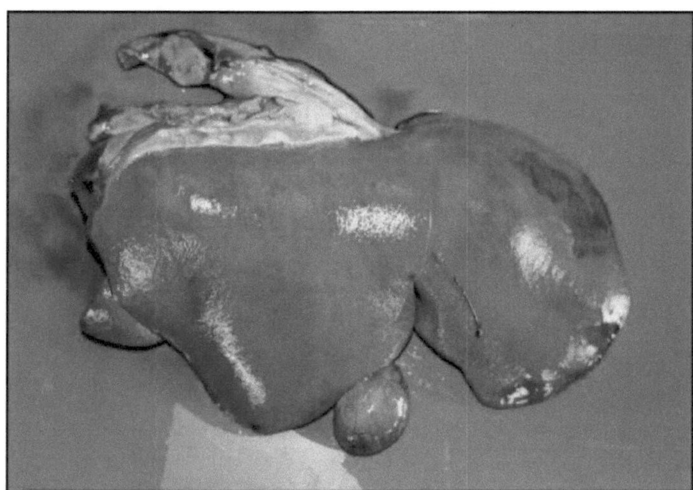

Figure 28 - Figado aumentado de volume, com bordas arredondadas, coloração amarelada e vesicula biliar cheia de ovino com intoxicação chónico experimental por cobre.

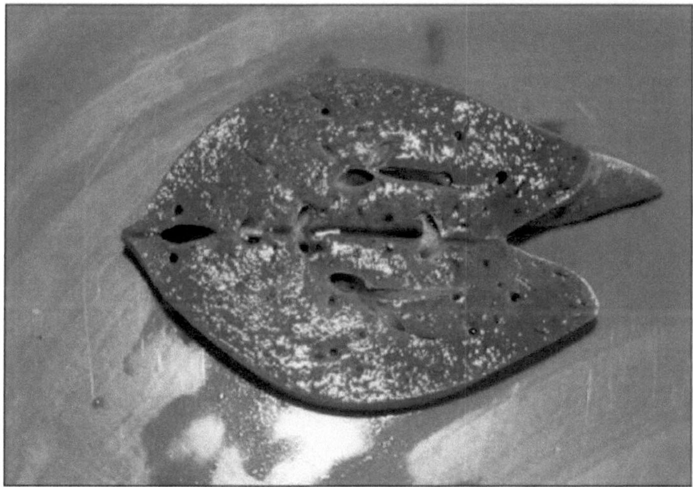

Figure 29 - Cut surface of liver (Figure 28) from sheep with chronic experimental copper intoxication.

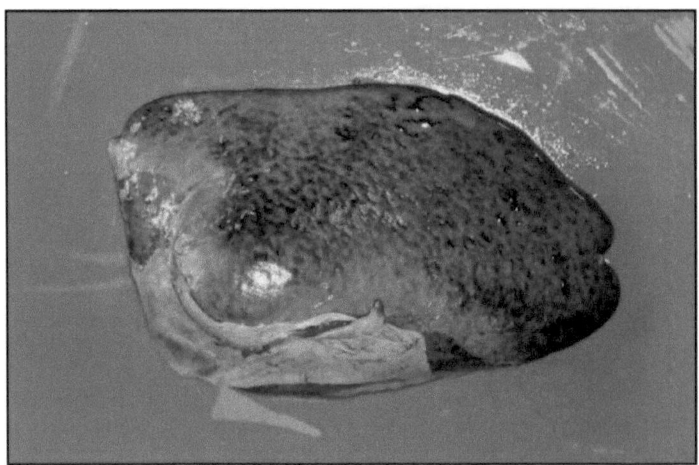

Figure 30 - Enlarged spleen with rounded edges in sheep with chronic experimental copper poisoning.

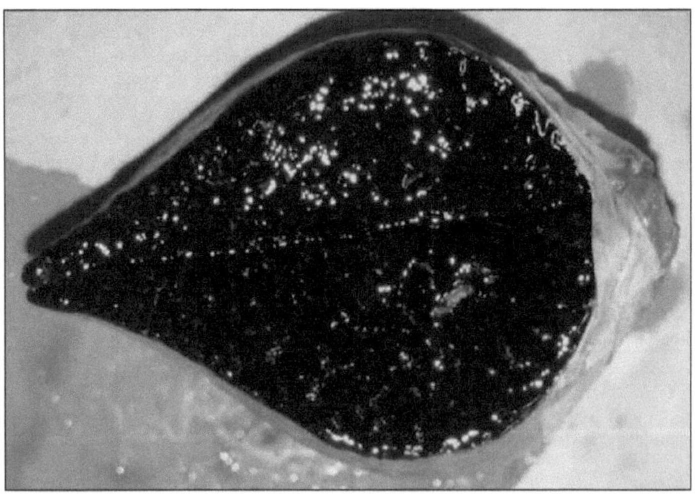

Figure 31 - Hyperemia on the cut surface of the spleen (Figure 30) of sheep with chronic experimental copper poisoning.

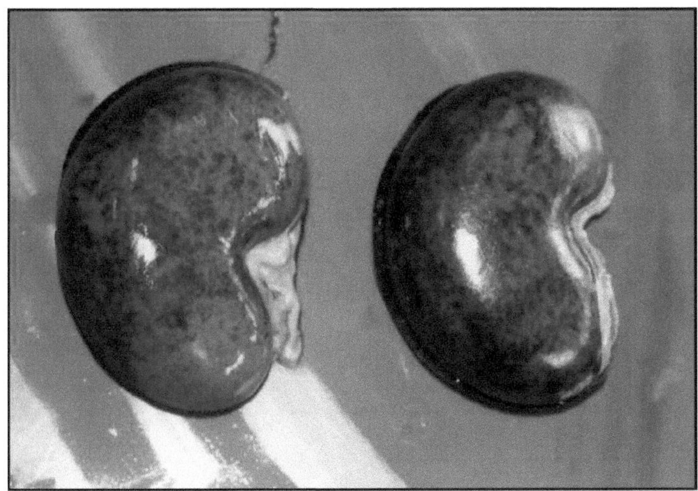

Figure 32 - Enlarged kidneys with blackened spots in the renal parenchyma of sheep with chronic experimental copper poisoning.

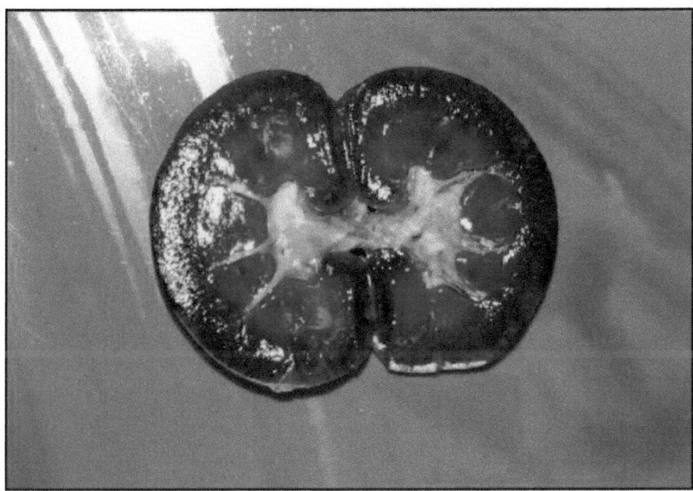

Figure 33 - Enlarged kidney with blackened cortical region and yellowish renal pelvis in sheep with chronic experimental copper poisoning.

5.8.2.   Histopathological findings

Microscopic alterations were found in the livers, kidneys and spleens of the animals experimentally intoxicated with copper. Other organs such as the heart, bladder, intestines, adrenal glands, pre-stomach, eyes, skeletal muscles and central nervous system showed no noteworthy changes. Histological sections of the liver showed disorganization of hepatocyte cords (Figures 34 and 39); presence of a multifocal, mild neutrophilic inflammatory infiltrate (Figures 35 and 36); megalocytosis, multifocal intrahepatic and extrahepatic cholestasis (Figures 37 and 38); necrosis of centrilobular hepatocytes The animals' spleens showed diffuse and marked congestion of red pulp, and microscopy of the kidneys showed degeneration of the cortical renal tubules, with the presence of reddish and brownish pigment in the cytoplasm, presence of a marked amount of red blood cells in the lumen of cortical renal tubules, multifocal lymphocytic inflammatory infiltrate in the interstitium, diffuse and moderate congestion of blood vessels, mild multifocal glomerular edema and multifocal and moderate calcification of medullary renal tubules.

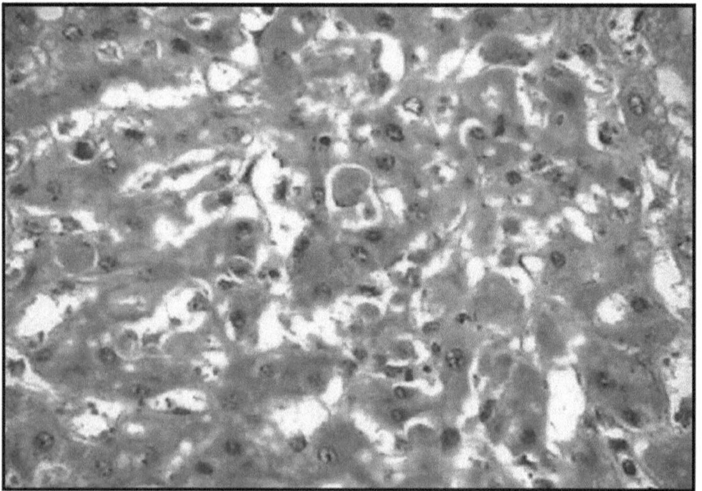

Figure 34 - Photomicrograph of liver, showing disorganization of hepatocyte cords in sheep with chronic experimental copper poisoning. 10x. HE.

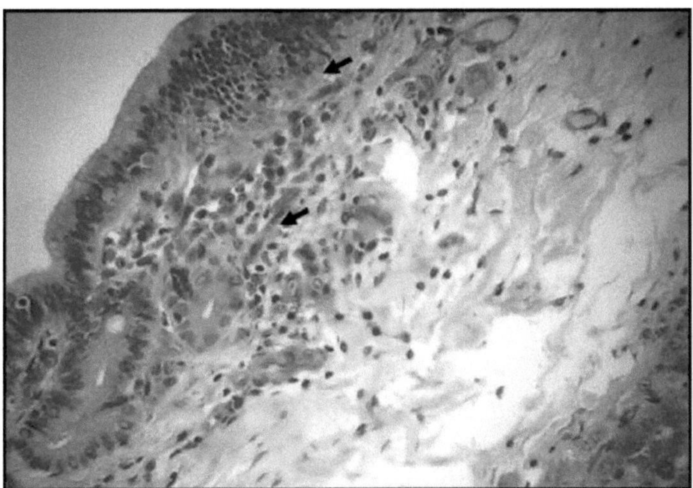

Figura 35 - Photomicrograph of gallbladder showing edema and lymphocytic inflammatory infiltrate (arrows) in the submucosa of the gallbladder of sheep with chronic experimental copper intoxication. 10x. HE.

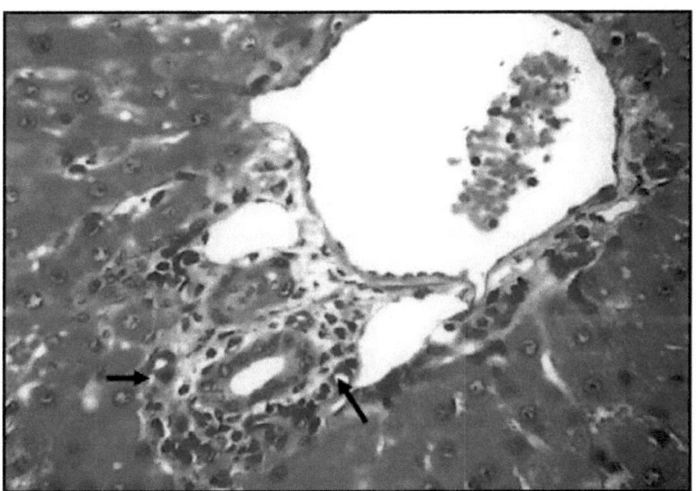

Figura 36 - Photomicrograph of liver showing periportal lymphocytic inflammatory infiltrate (arrows) from sheep with chronic experimental copper poisoning. 20x. HE.

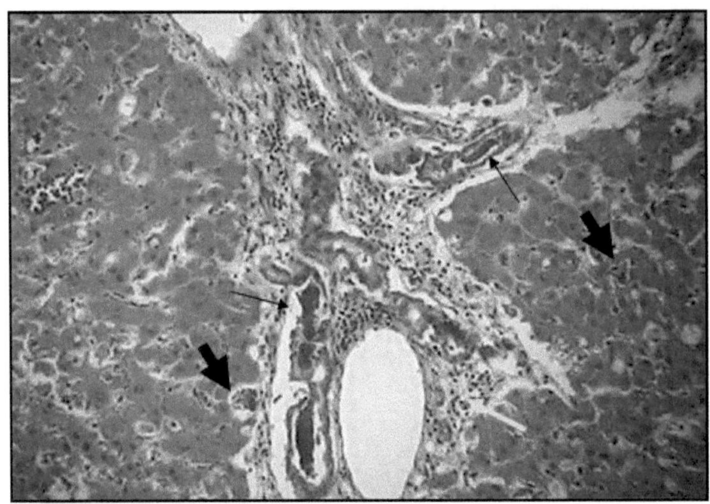

Figura 37 - Photomicrograph of liver showing periportal infiltrate (yellow arrow) and marked extrahepatic (thin arrow) and intrahepatic (wide arrow) cholestasis in sheep with chronic experimental copper poisoning. 4x. HE.

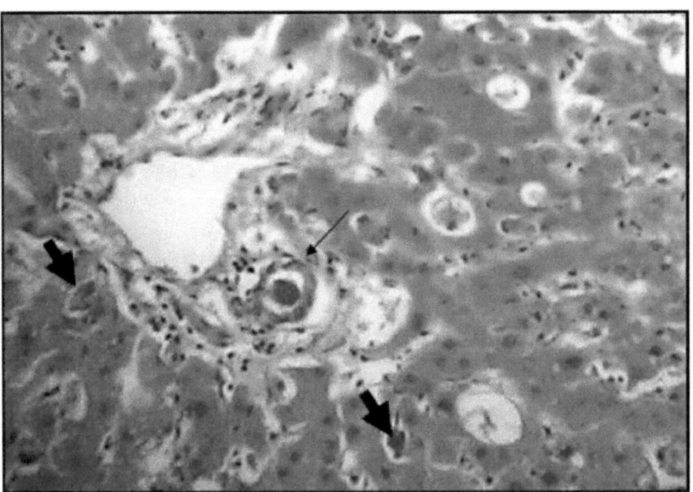

Figura 38 - Photomicrograph of the liver showing extrahepatic (thin arrow) and intrahepatic (wide arrow) cholestasis in sheep with chronic experimental copper poisoning.10x. HE.

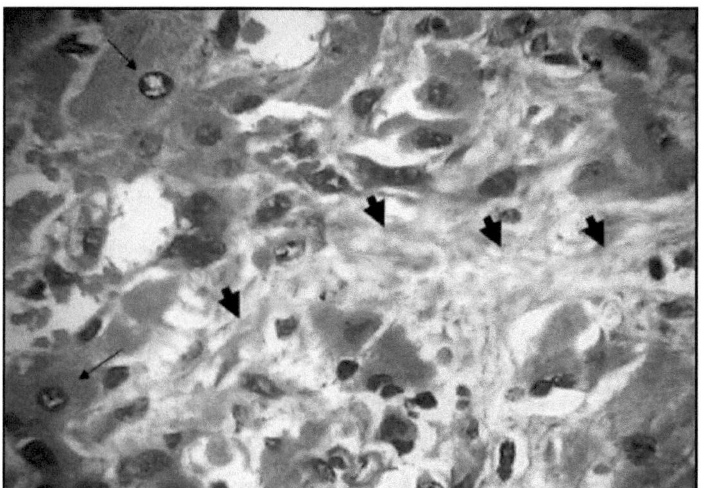

Figura 39 - Photomicrograph of liver showing disorganization of hepatocyte chordae, megalocytosis (thin arrow) and areas of hepatocyte necrosis (wide arrow) in sheep with chronic experimental copper poisoning. 40x. HE.

6. DISCUSSION

According to work carried out by ORTOLANI (1996), MACHADO (1998) and SOARES (2004), chronic copper poisoning in sheep has a pre-hemolytic and hemolytic phase, and during the pre-hemolytic phase, without relevant information in the animal's history, clinical diagnosis is extremely difficult.

The experimental protocol proposed by MACHADO (1998) and used in this study was highly effective in triggering the hemolytic phase. However, the total amount of copper sulphate given to the G-2 animals was high when compared to the results found by MACHADO (1998) and SOARES (2004). The probable explanation for this difference lies in the racial pattern of the animals, since MACHADO (2008) used crossbred animals (½ Sulfok blood x ½ Crioulo blood) and SOARES (2004) Santa Inês sheep, while in the present study the animals were of no defined breed. These results strengthen the premise that some sheep breeds, such as the Sulfok and Texel, are more susceptible to intoxication than the Scotish Blackface, Merino and Welch, and that this predisposition is directly related to a greater ability to absorb dietary copper and subsequently retain it in the liver (ORTOLANI, 1996).

After hepatic saturation and the release of copper into the plasma, significant damage occurs to the erythrocyte membranes, culminating in hemolytic anemia, causing a reduction of 60% of the initial erythrocyte values. The elimination of hemoglobin through the urine induces macroscopic hemoglobinuria, leading to acute tubular necrosis, so even if the sheep recover from the anemia, they can develop acute renal failure, leading to death (ORTOLANI, 1996). However, it is worth noting that before the onset of the hemolytic crisis, the animals show clinical signs such as apathy, inappetence and anorexia. The timing of these clinical signs was similar to those obtained by ORTOLANI et al. (2003), while SOARES (2004) noted the appearance of diarrhea with mucus and anorexia around four and two days before the hemolytic crisis, respectively. The presence of the clinical signs shown in this study associated with a comparable history of intoxication would indicate the start of preventive treatment for the hemolytic crisis.

As the hemolytic crisis develops, the animal's clinical condition worsens rapidly. At this point, the clinical signs presented by the G-2 sheep were similar to those reported by ROUBIES et al. (2008). On the day of the crisis, there is a drop in the number of red blood cells, affecting the transport of oxygen and nutrients needed to maintain body homeostasis, causing the animals to show marked apathy and dyspnea. In addition to these signs, the presence of chocolatey mucous membranes was very common.

MACHADO (1998) observed chocolate-colored mucous membranes until the third day after the hemolytic crisis, after which the mucous membranes became icteric. According to JAIN (1993), the observation of chocolatey mucous membranes is due to the presence of methemoglobin.

Due to hemolysis, there were significant changes in the blood counts of the animals in G-2, when compared to those in G-1 and the moments before M4. Thus, the number of red blood cells decreased by approximately 50% over the course of 48 hours after the detection of the hemolytic crisis. Similar results were obtained by MACHADO (1998), ORTOLANI (2003), SOARES (2004) and ROUBIES (2008). The reduction in the number of red blood cells associated with the hemolytic process led to a significant reduction in the hematocrit and hemoglobin values.

With regard to erythrocyte morphology, it can be seen that from M0 to M3 there was a predominance of red blood cells with a discoid pattern and around 15% in the form of macrocytes, kinizocytes and dacryocytes. According to JAIN (1993) and FELDMAN (2000), the presence of dacryocytes is due to changes in the protein cytoskeleton of red blood cells due to deforming events. These alterations are mainly observed in anemias associated with the presence of Heinz bodies, thalassemias and myelofibrosis. Macrocytes represent morphologically normal erythrocytes with a mean corpuscular volume above normal, while kinizocytes comprise red blood cells with a central band of hemoglobin, forming two free spaces on the surface of the red blood cells, creating the appearance of a truncated cell. Although this type of cell is associated with anemia in humans and dogs (FELDMAN, 2000), in the present study the finding of a low percentage of these cells in both G-1 and G-2 suggests that morphological changes may be present due to metabolism and constant erythrocyte renewal.

The mechanisms that promote morphological changes in red blood cell membranes have not been fully elucidated. The mechanism of hemolysis promoted by copper intoxication is not well understood. According to JAIN (1993) and INABA (2000), the cytotoxic effects occur due to the interaction of copper with the sulfhydryl groups of the erythrocyte membrane proteins and the lipid peroxidation of the membranes, generating in this process the formation of oxidizing agents, in addition to the inhibition of important enzymes for red blood cells such as glutathione reductase, 6-glucose-D-phosphate and pyruvate kinase, causing inhibition of cellular oxidative metabolism, allowing copper to damage the erythrocyte membrane, altering its morphology and generating a hemolytic condition. However, based on studies by SOARES (2004), it can be said that all damage to the erythrocyte membrane is related to alterations in the erythrocyte oxidative metabolism generated by copper.

The erythrocyte pattern at times M4 to M6 was marked by the presence of acanthocytes, which are spiculated erythrocytes with severe projections on their surface. Their presence is due to alterations in the phospholipids in the erythrocyte membrane, and they are generally associated with the presence of diffuse liver diseases and diets with high levels of cholesterol. According to SOARES (2004), during the hemolytic crisis there is a decrease in the amount of reduced erythrocyte glutathione and an increase in serum malonyldialdehyde levels, confirming the presence of oxidative damage to erythrocytes and other tissues. Stomatocytes are related to the presence of obstructive liver disease and associated with chronic anemia in dogs. Codocytes, commonly called target cells, are erythrocytes with a dense central area of hemoglobin, due to alterations in the cell membrane or a decrease in cell hemoglobin levels, or both. They are found in hypochromic anemia and in liver diseases that lead to cholestasis (FELDMAN, 2000).

In addition to acanthocytes and codocytes, keratocytes were found, which are irregular erythrocytes with spicules and are related to the presence of disseminated intravascular coagulation, microangiohepatic hemolytic anemia and renal failure. The presence of Heinz corpuscles was noted 48 hours after the hemolytic crisis.

During the hemolytic crisis, the animals in G-2 showed leucocytosis with neutrophilia and lymphocytes within the values established for the species (PUGH, 2005); however, the lymphocytes were fewer when compared to G-1. These findings corroborate those of MÉNDEZ (2001).

The enzyme gamma glutamyltransferase was an excellent indicator of chronic copper intoxication in the G-2 sheep, since its activity began to increase 30 days before the onset of the hemolytic crisis (M1), with more intense activity at times M2 and M3 of the experimental intoxication. With the onset of the hemolytic crisis, its activity was even greater. Similar results were found by MACHADO (1998), AUZA, et al., (1999) and MÉNDEZ (2001), who found that GGT activity rose around 28 days before the onset of the hemolytic crisis. LEMOS et al. (1997) also found increases in GGT levels, however, these increases were identified 21 days before the onset of clinical changes. The possible explanation for an early increase in GGT may be related to compression of the bile ducts due to liver congestion.

With regard to AST, while MACHADO (1998) obtained significant increases in the activity of this enzyme 14 days before the hemolytic crisis, in this study the increase in AST activity was noted seven days before the clinical manifestation of experimental intoxication (M3), with serum activity exceeding 300 U/L. UNDERWOOD & SUTTLE (2001), reported that the AST enzyme is an excellent indicator of cupric intoxication, however it can be seen in this study that GGT activity showed an earlier increase. Although GGT is an early indicator of copper intoxication, increases in AST can more accurately indicate the onset of the hemolytic crisis, since this enzyme indicates the presence of liver necrosis (TENNANT, 1997).

With regard to serum CK activity, it was clear that its kinetics in both G-1 and G-2 sheep remained the same up to M4. At M5 and M6, there was a significant increase in CK serum activity in G2 sheep. The increase in serum CK activity at M5 and M6 may be related to the intoxicated sheep's lying down, which causes muscle damage.

Serum total protein levels remained similar between G-1 and G-2 sheep during all phases of chronic copper intoxication. Polyacrylamide gel electrophoresis showed the behavior of some proteins during the different stages of intoxication. Among these proteins, ceruloplasmin, transferrin, the 35,000 Da protein and light chain IgG were the ones that showed marked alterations during intoxication.

Ceruloplasmin showed a reduction in serum levels in G2 sheep from M1 to M4, when compared to baseline values, and at M5 (24 hours after the hemolytic crisis) its activity increased by 37%. FLORIS et al. (2000) describe that human patients with Wilson's disease (chronic copper poisoning) have reduced or undetectable circulating levels of ceruloplasmin. The increase in ceruloplasmin observed in M5 is due to the fact that ceruloplasmin is an acute phase protein and responds to the inflammatory process triggered by hemolysis. GUTTERIDGE et al. (1980) reported that ceruloplasmin acts as an important antioxidant, inhibiting lipid peroxidation processes much more potently than superoxide dismutase and catalase. Thus, during the hemolytic crisis, ceruloplasmin plays a role in cellular protection against free radicals, corroborating the work of SOARES (2004) who found the presence of greater antioxidant activity during the height of the hemolytic crisis.

Transferrin is a negative acute phase protein whose serum levels tend to decrease in the presence of inflammatory conditions (KANEKO, 1997). However, in this study, this protein was found to be highly active in G-2 sheep between moments M1 and M6 of cumulative cupric intoxication, with its maximum increase at M2, when it reached 126% compared to M0. The increase in transferrin at M2 coincided with the moment when there was the greatest reduction in serum ceruloplasmin in the G-2 sheep. At M4, transferrin increased by 76% in G-2 sheep. The increase in serum transferrin levels may be associated with liver damage (KANEKO, 1997) related to copper accumulation.

The increase in light chain IgG, especially at time point M4, may be related to both liver damage and the hemolytic anemia present (KANEKO, 1997). The 35,000 Da protein was elevated during moments M1 to M6 of cumulative copper intoxication, with a 328% increase in its activity at M2.

The clinical pathological picture as well as the morphological changes in the erythrocytes were directly influenced by the amount of copper released, in addition to the individual response of the animals.

Copper was released into the bloodstream at M4 in the G-2 sheep. However, it was noted that the G-2 animals had significantly higher serum copper levels than the G-1 sheep at times M2 and M3, although this was within the limits established for the species. At time point M4, serum copper levels rose significantly and at times M5 and M6 these values were lower than at time point M4, although they remained high.

The biochemical findings associated with the alterations obtained in the serum proteinogram suggest that liver damage began at M2, with a period of 15 days for complete saturation of the hepatocytes and release of copper into the circulatory system.

Necropsy of the intoxicated animals revealed generalized jaundice, a friable yellowish liver, dark brown kidneys and brownish urine. Liver histopathology showed enlarged, pleomorphic hepatocytes with vacuoles of various sizes in their cytoplasm and intra- and extra-hepatic cholestasis, corroborating the work of BOSTWICK (1982), RIET-CORREA et al. (1989), LEMOS, et al. (1997), MÉNDEZ, (2001) and ROUBIES et al. (2008) The disorganization of the hepatocyte cords and the presence of a periportal lymphocytic inflammatory infiltrate were not found in other studies.

7. CONCLUSION

This work has led to the conclusion that:

- The experimental model used proved to be effective;

- The GGT enzyme was shown to be an early indicator of cumulative copper intoxication;

- Serum ceruloplasmin levels were decreased and transferrin, 35,000 Da protein and light chain IgG levels were increased 15 days before the hemolytic crisis;

- The main clinical signs of the intoxicated animals were: anorexia, yellowish mucous membranes, soft, dark green feces and hemoglobinuria;

- During the hemolytic crisis, the intoxicated sheep presented a picture of macrocytic normochromic anemia associated with neutrophilic leukocytosis, elevated serum AST and GGT levels, predominantly red blood cells with acanthocyte morphology and hypercupremia;

- The main necropsy findings are characterized by yellowish mucous membranes, liver and other tissues, blackened kidneys and brownish urine;

- The main histological changes in the liver of intoxicated animals were: hepatocyte megalocytosis, hepatocyte cord disorganization, intra- and extrahepatic cholestasis and peri-portal lymphocytic inflammatory infiltrate.

8. BIBLIOGRAPHICAL REFERENCES

AUZA, N. J.; OLSON, W. G.; MURPHY, M. J.; LINN, J. G. Diagnosis and treatment of copper toxicosis in ruminants. **J. Am. Vet. Med. Assoc.**, v. 214, n. 11, p. 1624 - 1628, 1999.

BOSTWICK, J. L. Copper toxicosis in sheep **J. Am. Vet. Med. Assoc.**, v. 180, n. 4, p. 386 - 387, 1982.

BRADBERRY, S. Copper. **Medicine**, v. 35, n. 11, p. 608, 2007.

FLORIS, G.; MEDDA, R.; PADIGLIA, A.; MUSCI, G. The physiopathological significance of ceruloplasmin/ a possible therapeutic approach. Bio. Pharm., v. 60, p. 1735 - 1741, 2000.

GONZALEZ, F. H. D.; BARCELLOS, J.; PATINO, H. O.; **Metabolic profile in ruminants: its use in nutrition and nutritional diseases**. Porto Alegre: Gràfica UFRGS. 2000. 438p.

GOONERATNE, S.R., BUCKLEY, W.T., CHRISTENSEN, D.A. Rewiew of copper deficiency and metabolism in ruminants. **Can. J. Anim. Sci.,** v.69, p.819-845, 1989.

GUTTERIDGE, J. M. C.; RICHMOND, R.; HALLIWELL, B. Oxygen free-radicals and lipid peroxidation: inhibition by the protein caeruloplasmin. **Febs Letters**. v. 112, n. 2, p. 269 - 271, 1980.

HUMANN-ZIEHANK, E.; BICKHARDT, K. Effects of d-penicillamine on urinary copper excretion in high-copper supplemented sheep. **J. Vet. Med. A. Physiol. Pathol. Clin. Med.**, v. 48, n. 9, p.537-544, 2001.

HUMPHRIES, W. R.; MORRICE, P. C.; BREMNER, I. A convenient method for the treatment of chronic copper poisoning in sheep using subcutaneous ammonium tetrathiomolybdate. **Vet. Rec.**, v. 123, n. 2, p. 51-53, jul.1988.

INABA, M. Red blood cell membrane defects. In: FELDMAN, B. F.; JOSEPH, G. Z.; JAIN, N. C. **Schalm's Veterinary Hematology**, 5. ed. Canada: Lippincot Williams & Wilkins, 2000. p. 1012 - 1020.

JAIN, N. C. **Essentials of veterinary hematology**. Philadelphia: Lea & Febiger, 1993. 417p.

KANEKO, J. J. Serum proteins and the dysproteinemias. In: KANEKO, J. J.; HARVEY, J. W.; BRUSS, M. L. **Clinical biochemistry of domestic animals.** 5 ed. San Diego: Academic Press, 1997, chap. 5, p. 117 - 138.

KARGIN, F.; SEYREK, K.; BILDIK, A.; AYPAK, S. Determination of the levels of zinc, copper, calcium, phosphorus and magnesium of chios ewes in the Aydin region. **Turk. J. Vet. Anim. Sci.**, v 28 p. 609 -612, 2004.

KOWALCZYK, T.; POPE, A. L.; BERGER, K. C.; MUGGENBURG, B. A. Chronic copper toxicosis in sheep fed dry feed. **J. Am. Vet. Med. Assoc.**, v. 145, n. 4, p. 352 - 358, aug. 1964.

LAEMMLI, U. K. Cleavage of structural proteins during the assembly of the head of bacteriophage T4. **Nature.** v. 227, p. 680 - 685, 1970.

LEMOS, R. A. A.; RANGEL, J. M. R. R.; OSÓRIO, A. L. A. R.; MORAES, S. S.; NAKAZATO, L.; SALVADOR, S.C.; MARTINS, S. Clinical, pathological and laboratory changes in chronic copper intoxication in sheep. **Ciência Rural,** v. 27, n. 3, p. 457 - 463, 1997.

LUNA, L. G. **Manual of histologic stauning methods of the armed forces institute of pathology**. 3 ed., New York: McGraw-hill, 1968, 258p.

MACHADO, C. H. **Use of tetrathiomolybdate in the treatment of experimental cupric intoxication in sheep: clinical and toxicological evaluation.** Sâo Paulo, 1998, 138.f. (Doctorate in Veterinary Medicine) Faculty of Veterinary Medicine and Zootechny, University of Sâo Paulo. Sâo Paulo, 1998.

MCDOWELL, L. R. **Minerals in animal and human nutrition**. San Diego: Academic Press, 1992. 524p.

MÉNDEZ, M. C. Chronic copper poisoning. In: RIET-CORREA, F.; SCHIELD, A. C.; MÉNDEZ, M. C. **Doenças de Ruminantes e Eqüinos**. v. 1. Sâo Paulo: Livraria Varela, 2001, chap. 2,. p.181-186.

MILTIMORE, J.E., MASON, J.L. Cooper to molybdenun ratio and molybdenun and copper concentration in ruminant feeds. **Can. J. Anim. Sci.,** v.51, p.193 - 200, 1971.

ORTOLANI, E. L. Intoxications and metabolic diseases in sheep: copper intoxication, urolithiasis and pregnancy toxemia. In: SOBRINHO, A. G.; BATISTA, A. M. V.; SIQUEIRA, E. R.; ORTOLANI, E. L.; SUSIN, I.; SILVA, J. I. C.; TEIXEIRA, J. C.; BORBA, M. F. S. **Nutriçao de Ovinos**. Jaboticabal: Funep, 1996. p. 241 - 258.

ORTOLANI, E. L. Macro and microelements. In: SPINOSA, H. S.; GORNIAK, S. L.; BERNADI, M. M. **Farmacologia Aplicada à Medicina Veterinària**. Rio de Janeiro: Guanabara Koogan, 2002. p. 641-651.

ORTOLANI, E. L.; MACHADO, C. H.; SUCUPIRA, M. C. A. Assessment of some clinical and laboratory variables for early diagnosis of cumulative copper poisoning in sheep. **Vet. Human. Toxicol.**, v. 45, n. 6, p. 289 - 293, 2003.

PUGH, D. G. **Clinica de ovinos e caprinos**. Sâo Paulo: Roca, 2005, 513 p.

RADOSTITS, O. M.; MAYHEW, I. G. J.; HOUSTON, D. M. **Clinica veterinària: um tratado de doenças dos bovinos, ovinos, suinos, caprinos e equinos.** 9 ed. Rio de Janeiro: Guanabara Koogan, 2002. 1747 p.

RIET-CORREA, F.; OLIVEIRA, J. A.; MENDEZ, M. C. Chronic copper poisoning in sheep in Rio Grande do Sul. **Pesq. Vet. Bras.**,. v. 9, n. 3/ 4, p. 51-54, 1989.

ROUBIES, N.; GIADINIS, N. D.; POLIZOPOULOU, Z.; ARGIROUDIS, S. A retrospective study of chronic copper poisoning in 79 sheep flocks in Greece (1987 - 2007). **J. Vet. Pharmacol. Therap.**, n. 31, p. 181 - 183, 2008.

SANSINANEA, A. S.; CERONE,S. I.; ELPERDING, A.; AUZA, N. Glucose-6-phosphate dehydrogenase activity in erythrocytes from chronically copper-poisoned sheep. **Comp. Biochem. Physiol.**, v. 114C, n. 3, p. 197-200, 1996.

SMITH, B. P. **Treatise on Large Animal Veterinary Internal Medicine.** Sao Paulo: Manole, 3. ed., 2006.

SOARES, P. C. **Efeitos da intoxicação cúprica e do tratamento com tetratiomolibdato sobre a função renal e o metabolismo oxidativo de ovinos**. Sao Paulo, 2004, 117.f. (Doctorate in Veterinary Medicine) Faculty of Veterinary Medicine and Zootechny, University of Sao Paulo. Sao Paulo, 2004.

TENNANT, B. C. Hepatic function. In: KANEKO, J. J.; HARVEY, J. W.; BRUSS, M. L. **Clinical biochemistry of domestic animals.** 5 ed. San Diego: Academic Press, 1997, chap. 13, p. 327-349.

TURK, J. R.; CASTEEL, S. W. Clinical biochemistry in toxicology. In: KANEKO, J. J.; HARVEY, J. W.; BRUSS, M. L. **Clinical biochemistry of domestic animals.** 5 ed. San Diego: Academic Press, 1997, chap. 28, p. 829-832.

THRALL, M. A. **Hematology and clinical veterinary biochemistry**. Sao Paulo: Roca, 2007, 582p.

UNDERWOOD, E. J.; SUTTLE, N. F. **The Mineral Nutrition of Livestock**. 3 ed. Wallingford: Cabi Publishing, 2001. 614 p.

VIEIRA, S. **Introduçâo à bioestatistica**. 3 ed. Rio de Janeiro: Editora Campus, 1998. 196p.

ZHANG, Y.; LI, B.; CHEN, C.; GAO, Z. Hepatic distribution of iron, copper, zinc and cadmium- containing proteins in normal and iron overload. **Biometals**. Available at: < http://www.springerlink.com/content/j2r366022l7kt481/> Accessed: September 2008.

55

APPENDIX 1

Table 16 - Bromatological composition of the Tifton grass hay and concentrated feed given to the sheep during the experiment.

Bromatological composition-	Food	
	Hay	Concentrate
Dry matter (%)	88,25	89,34
Mineral matter (%)	4,75	17,81
Crude Protein (%)	5,25	9,43
Crude fiber (%)	34,25	20,10
Ethereal extract (%)	1,78	1,52
Non-nitrogenous extractive matter (%)	53,98	51,16
Calcium (%)	0,47	1,56
Phosphorus (%)	0,21	0,34
Sulphur (%)	0,15	0,19
Copper (ppm)	5,0	7,0
Molybdenum (ppm)	1,15	0,30

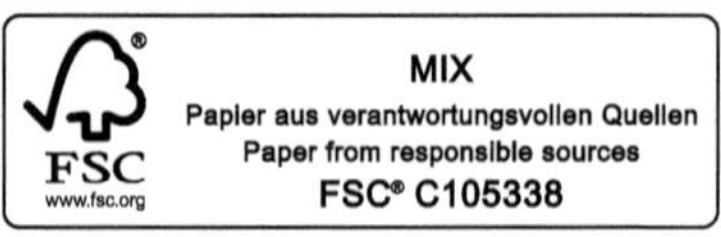

Printed by Books on Demand GmbH, Norderstedt / Germany